"*Hypnotize Yourself Out of Pain No*  strategies in the management of pain, o and well-grounded approaches that re Dr. Eimer permits readers to become at their own pace. Readers learn to: assess their progress through a variety of rating sheets, engage in self-hypnosis, use soothing mind-body interventions and exercises—all to generate pain relief now. This book promises to be of great value for anyone determined to change pain behaviors into well behaviors but also represents a tremendous resource to any health-care professional assisting patients in managing pain."

—*Elvira V. Lang, M.D., Associate Professor of Radiology and Medicine, Harvard Medical School Director, Cardiovascular and Interventional Radiology at Beth Israel Deaconess Medical Center, Boston*

"A valuable and effective self-help manual for coping with pain—one of the best documented applications of therapeutic hypnosis."

—*Ernest Rossi, Ph.D., author of* The Psychobiology of Mind-Body Healing: New Concepts of Therapeutic Hypnosis

"A thought-provoking book for the person who suffers from chronic pain. Great reading for both the layperson and professional."

—*Charles B. Mutter, M.D., ABMH, psychiatrist in private practice, Past President, American Society of Clinical Hypnosis Diplomate, and Past President, American Board of Medical Hypnosis*

"A valuable and much needed text detailing many hypnotic approaches to the treatment of pain. Among them, Dr. Eimer employs Ego State Therapy in a responsible and innovative way."

—*John G. Watkins, Ph.D., Professor Emeritus of Psychology, University of Montana, Missoula and Helen H. Watkins, M.A., Licensed Clinical Psychologist, authors of* Ego States: Theory and Therapy *and founders of Ego State Therapy*

"This book has much to offer the person with persistent pain. Dr. Eimer goes right to the questions that need to be answered for a satisfactory understanding of persistent pain, taking into account the coping style of the person who has it. His search for relief from the pain of his own physical illness has led him to research and practice the self-hypnotic skills that have helped keep him from being an invalid. He has condensed this research into a book that is a summary of the best ways to achieve pain relief with self-hypnosis."

—Dabney M. Ewin, M.D., FACS, ABMH, Diplomate, American Board of Medical Hypnosis and Past President, American Society of Clinical Hypnosis

"Absolutely an excellent resource for both therapists and for those who experience chronic pain. The suggestions and exercises provide a great variety of ideas for the novice and the experienced practitioner alike. This is an excellent book."

—Dr Susi Strang Wood MBChB, MRCGP, UKCP Psychotherapist

—Craig N Wood MSc, MH(Acc), UKCP Psychotherapist

"*Hypnotize Yourself Out of Pain Now!* is described as a "powerful, user-friendly program for anyone searching for immediate pain relief", and it is all of this. It is also the most comprehensive and effective program for lasting pain relief that I have ever found.

Bruce Eimer combines over 20 years of knowledge, skills and experience, with the empathy and understanding of someone who has developed these effective methods through learning to manage his own chronic pain.

Those who suffer chronic pain have often spent a long time trying medical and alternative approaches without finding relief, and under such circumstances, it is understandable to lose hope and motivation to keep trying new methods. If this describes you, take heart – reading this book will really make a difference for you and will help you regain control of your mind and body.

If you are a professional working with those in pain, this book offers ways and means to help each individual using the combination of methods that will suit them best.

Bruce Eimer offers straightforward, honest, caring support alongside all the information, practical methods and different approaches you might need to reduce any kind of pain to manageable levels."

*—Susanna Bellini, NLP trainer, counsellor, hypnotherapist and also a chronic pain survivor.*

"This book is valuable and thought-provoking for people experiencing chronic pain. Eimer approaches his subject with the first-hand knowledge and commitment of someone who, after an accident, sought relief from the resulting persistent pain. Not wanting to remain an invalid, he summarises the techniques which freed him.

Principally directed at the layperson, this book will also prove a resource for the healthcare professional helping patients manage their pain.

"...to tame pain, we must use our brain": we are aided to solve the puzzle of pain, separating the sensory, cognitive and emotional experiences of pain which keep chronic sufferers in a vicious cycle. Techniques are explored to evaluate, then practice self-hypnosis to reduce the everyday impact of pain and live with it in a meaningful manner. Hypnosis is introduced in a way which allows readers to choose the induction method which best suits them. Self-suggestion is explained so that readers feel unthreatened by the process.

The penultimate chapter is entitled Become AWARE and find your inner balance. The acronym AWARE – Accept the pain, Watch your experience, Act functionally, Remove yourself from pain, and Expect the best – gives a clear idea of the positive self-change which Eimer hopes sufferers can achieve on their journey."

ANTHONY SCRATCHLEY is a Hazelden-trained counsellor, with some years in practice. He has also worked in sports management.

*—Anthony Scratchley, Addiction Today Magazine*

"Although written as a self-help manual, *Hypnotize Yourself Out of Pain Now!* is a fantastic resource for practising therapists as well as for anyone suffering from chronic pain themselves.

With so many self-hypnosis books currently on the market, this excellent account distinguishes itself by being clearly focused on a particular problem and written by someone who is not only a clinical psychologist, but who has himself suffered from chronic pain.

Bruce Eimer was injured in a major road accident in 1993, giving him first-hand experience of what his patients had been going through. As a result he pledged that he 'would do anything within his power to help other chronic pain sufferers cope'.

This experience gives the book a degree of commitment, focus and personal investment that should serve in itself to inspire and encourage fellow sufferers, as well as convince them of the benefits of hypnosis.

Because pain has both a sensory and an emotional content, Dr Eimer believes it is ideally suited to the kinds of relaxation, cognitive and imaginative techniques employed in the therapeutic use of hypnosis.

The book is absolutely bursting with practical self-help exercises which avoid overwhelming the reader by being contained within the framework of a clearly structured programme of self-treatment.

Having first offered information to assist in understanding 'the puzzle of pain', Dr Eimer provides comprehensive questionnaires which allow the reader to evaluate their own experience of pain.

A clear explanation is given of the basics of hypnosis followed by an account of the benefits of self-hypnosis and how this in itself can help to alleviate discomfort.

The reader is then able to select from the huge range of coping strategies that form the core of the book. These are brought together in a step-by-step approach combining self-hypnosis, coping exercises and the use of self-suggestion.

The book culminates by offering detailed scripts that can be used to probe more deeply into the underlying causes of pain.

This is both an accessible and exceptionally thorough guide which is not just a very good aid to pain-relief, but also one of the most lucid introductions around to the therapeutic uses of hypnosis in the treatment of everyday problems."

—Julian Gill, Hypnotherapist, www.aspiretherapyonline.com

"Full of valuable information and empowering methods easily understood and practiced without any additional training, *Hypnotize Yourself Out of Pain Now!* provides the keys that can unlock solutions to even the most stubborn pain problems It's hard to imagine a better resource to the use of hypnosis with pain conditions. This book is a must for any pain library."

—Maggie Phillips, Ph.D., Author of Reversing Chronic Pain, Finding the Energy to Heal, and Healing the Divided Self.

"Bruce Eimer is a licensed clinical psychologist with more than twenty years experience in treating people with chronic pain. Now in its second edition, his remarkable self-help title paves the way for pain relief through self-hypnosis. Eimer shows how anyone can be their own healer by learning to hypnotize themselves out of pain and improving their relationship with themselves. With a number of powerful methods to reduce or eliminate discomfort and a free CD of exercises to assist in pain relief, this great value book and CD set will help anyone who is suffering to tap into their own innate ability to control and manage pain."

—Stephen Gawtry, Editor, The Watkins Review

"For anyone suffering from chronic pain, this book provides a thorough understanding of what pain is and how it presents itself and then what the reader can do to help themselves through the application of self-hypnosis. It is well structured, starting with an in depth explanation of the nature of pain that is dealt with in a manner that is accessible and clearly written. The second section leads the reader through various exercises that build skills in self-hypnosis and pain management. There are a number of methods for inducing hypnosis provided so that it should be possible for anyone to find something they can feel comfortable with and achieve positive results. This is also true of the strategies and suggestions available to the reader. The different questionnaires in the book allow the reader to measure their experience of pain and how that changes as they make progress. This makes it almost a workbook rather than simply a theoretical text on the subject.

The research for this book has obviously been extensive and Eimer evidences a comprehensive understanding of the field by providing copious references and a recommended further reading list.

This is an impressive work that will also provide a valuable reference for any professional working with clients with chronic pain."

*—Stuart Harragan, Clinical Hypnotherapist. Find out more about Harragan Hypnotherapy at www.harragan.org.uk*

# Hypnotize Yourself Out of Pain Now!

*Second Edition*

A Powerful, User-Friendly
Program for Anyone Searching
for Immediate Pain Relief

## Bruce N. Eimer, PhD, ABPP

Crown House Publishing Limited
www.crownhouse.co.uk
www.chpus.com

First published by

Crown House Publishing Ltd
Crown Buildings, Bancyfelin, Carmarthen, Wales, SA33 5ND, UK
**www.crownhouse.co.uk**
and
Crown House Publishing Company LLC
6 Trowbridge Drive, Suite 5, Bethel, CT 06801 USA
**www.crownhousepublishing.com**

© 2008 Bruce N. Eimer. Reprinted 2009.

The right of Bruce N. Eimer to be identified as the author of this work
has been asserted by him in accordance with the Copyright, Designs and
Patents Act 1988.

First edition published by New Harbinger Publications, Inc. 2002
(Original ISBN: 1572242809)

All rights reserved. Except as permitted under current legislation no part
of this work may be photocopied, stored in a retrieval system, published,
performed in public, adapted, broadcast, transmitted, recorded or
reproduced in any form or by any means, without the prior permission
of the copyright owners. Enquiries should be addressed to Crown House
Publishing Limited.

**British Library of Cataloguing-in-Publication Data**
A catalogue entry for this book is available from the British Library.
International Standard Book Number
**10 digit ISBN 184590087-1**
**13 digit ISBN 978-184590087-8**

**Library of Congress Control Number**
**2007938977**
Printed and bound in the USA

*Bruce N. Eimer, Ph.D., A.B.P.P., is a licensed clinical psychologist in Philadelphia with more than twenty years of experience treating people with chronic pain using cognitive-behavioral and hypnosis strategies. Dr. Eimer is a Board Certified Diplomate of the American Board of Professional Psychology in the specialty of Cognitive-Behavioral Psychology, a Fellow of the American Society of Clinical Hypnosis, and an Approved Consultant in Clinical Hypnosis. He also holds board certifications in pain management and medical psychotherapy. He is a life member of the American Psychological Association and a member of the Society for Psychological Hypnosis and the Society for Clinical and Experimental Hypnosis. Dr. Eimer is a chronic pain survivor and has used self-hypnosis techniques to manage his own chronic pain.*

# Dedication

With gratitude and love to the memory of David B. Cheek, M.D., enlightened physician, generous teacher, caring therapist, supportive guide, hypnosis innovator, courageous explorer, creative and independent thinker, empathic healer, kind friend, and intuitive visionary into the light. Now an angel in heaven who continues to celebrate and champion life. 1912–1996

With gratitude and love to the memory of Helen Watkins, an empathic therapist and teacher, who taught me how to love my internal family. 1921–2002

With respect and love to the memory of Joe Eimer, my father, who lives on in me. May his blessed spirit continue to inspire noble resolves and acts of loving kindness. 1913–1996

"He who dwells in the secret place of the Most High Shall abide under the shadow of the Almighty." Psalm 91:1

# Contents

# Acknowledgments

In the years since I have joined the ranks of "people with pain," I have learned new information and developed new ideas about managing pain. I have grown personally. I have learned new coping skills and have tested them on myself. Having to find ways to deal with serious persistent pain has a way of pushing you!

Over the years, I have had the opportunity to learn and receive help from a number of wise people. I have read their writings and, in some cases, attended their seminars and workshops. I also have been graced with the opportunity to study personally with some of these individuals. I acknowledge these special people here.

David Cheek, M.D. encouraged me to write my first book, *Pain Management Psychotherapy* (Eimer and Freeman 1998), when it was just an idea. At that time, he reminded me that such a book was sorely needed. He helped me develop confidence in my ability to write from my heart and my head, and he convinced me of the importance of building on my own ideas.

When I was awaiting impending back surgery, Dr. Cheek worked with me on the telephone (he lived in California and I lived in Pennsylvania), employing helpful hypnotic techniques for reducing my anxiety and pain. He taught me how to use ideomotor movements and ideomotor finger signals (to be covered in chapter 8) to communicate with my unconscious mind. He helped me prepare my conscious and unconscious for the surgery. This alleviated a lot of my anxiety and imprinted in my unconscious positive expectations about all aspects of the experience. He "held my hand" over the telephone before my surgery, and he helped me go under general anesthesia with confidence that the outcomes of the surgery were going to be positive.

I met Dabney Ewin, M.D. before I became intimately acquainted with pain from a firsthand perspective. He taught me that good therapy is a whole lot more than a fifty-minute hour. He also personally taught me his hypno-analytic exploration and uncovering approaches to pain resolution. Over the years, Dr. Ewin has continued to be a mentor to me, a source of personal encouragement, wise guidance, inspiration, and new learning. He has been kind enough to write the foreword to this book. I also thank him for reading this manuscript in its various stages and offering helpful comments.

Among other things, Dr. Ewin has taught me that pain may be mandatory, but suffering is optional.

Jordan I. Zarren, M.S.W. is another dear friend who has changed my life. He is, at the time of this writing, the President-Elect of the American Society of Clinical Hypnosis. He is an exceptional clinical social worker and a master therapist and hypnosis clinician who has been using hypnosis for over forty years and who currently practices psychotherapy and clinical hypnosis in West Palm Beach, Florida.

Mr. Zarren is the originator of a unique approach to brief therapy that he calls "Brief Cognitive Hypnosis." I am grateful to him for teaching me his approach, generously mentoring me, and honoring me with the opportunity to help him write his clinical handbook, *Brief Cognitive Hypnosis: Facilitating the Change of Dysfunctional Behavior* (Zarren and Eimer 2001).

Jordan Zarren taught me how to use self-hypnosis. He taught me effective ways of communicating with my unconscious. He has been generous in granting me permission to use some of his material, and incorporate it into this work. I am also grateful to Mr. Zarren for reading this manuscript in its various stages and offering me helpfully honest comments.

I wish to acknowledge the late Frederick Evans, Ph.D., a past President of the International Society of Hypnosis, who was a clinical psychologist with the Pain Management Service of the Princeton Medical Center in New Jersey, and a thoughtful researcher, teacher, clinician, and contributor to clinical hypnosis and pain management psychology. I acknowledge Dr. Evans for having granted me permission to adapt some of his pain-assessment questions in chapter 2.

I wish to acknowledge Ronald Melzack, Ph.D. of McGill University, a research psychologist and luminary in the field of pain research. I am grateful to Dr. Melzack for granting me permission to reprint items from his widely used McGill Pain Questionnaire.

I wish to thank Jean Holroyd, Ph.D., a clinical and research psychologist at UCLA in Los Angeles and an eminent hypnosis practitioner and scholar, for the valuable feedback that she provided to me in the early stages of this project. I also wish to acknowledge Dr. Holroyd for the major contribution she has made to the field of hypnosis by creating, editing, and maintaining the hypnosis research database on the Internet. The Internet address for this Web site, which is supported by the American Society of Clinical Hypnosis (ASCH), is http://www.hypnosis-research.org/. It is a source for abstracts and citations of scientific research and clinical publications on hypnosis, and it also contains general information on hypnosis under "Hypnosis for the Seriously Curious."

I wish to acknowledge Dr. Devin J. Starlanyl, a dedicated physician and medical writer, for her tireless research directed at solving the puzzles of fibromyalgia and chronic myofascial pain syndrome and her persistent search for viable treatments for these complex pain syndromes. Her books are invaluable coping resources for all persons with chronic pain, and the health professionals who treat them. I am also indebted to Dr. Starlanyl for her valuable editorial feedback.

I am grateful to William Wester II, Ed.D., ABPH, Stuart Bassman, Ed.D., and to the American Society of Clinical Hypnosis Press for granting me permission to reprint Bassman and Wester's NO MORE PAIN acronym. I am especially grateful to Dr. Wester, a noted hypnosis scholar, clinical and forensic psychologist, author, professor, past President of the American Society of Clinical Hypnosis, and magician for his kind support and assurance that I was on the right track.

I am grateful to the following people for taking the time to read this manuscript before it became a real book and who offered their helpful editorial comments and kind suggestions: Charles Mutter, M.D., ABMH, a clinical and forensic psychiatrist, leading medical hypnotherapist, and past President of the American Society of Clinical Hypnosis; Alexander Levitan, M.D., ABMH, an internist, oncologist, leading medical hypnotherapist, author, and past President of the American Society of Clinical Hypnosis; and Helen Watkins, M.A. and John Watkins, Ph.D., a husband and wife clinical psychologist and hypnotherapy team who were the originators and codevelopers of Ego State Therapy, an innovative and powerful form of hypnotic therapy for inner conflict resolution and symptom reduction.

Melvin Gravitz, Ph.D., ABPH, a clinical and forensic psychologist, hypnotherapist, professor, and past President of the American Society of Clinical Hypnosis, is due many thanks for providing me with support, friendship, encouragement, editorial feedback, and guidance throughout this project.

Acknowledgments probably are also due others, but it's impossible to mention them all here.

I also acknowledge all of those persons in pain who, over the years as patients, have shared their stories with me. From them I have learned so much. I am grateful to these courageous individuals for granting me the privilege of listening to their stories and helping them manage their pain. Hopefully, some of the lessons I have learned in helping them escape from days of torture will continue to enable me to help others find comfort.

For the first edition, I also wish to thank my helpful managing and acquisitions editors at New Harbinger Publications, Catharine Sutker and Matthew McKay, Ph.D., for jumping on my initial ideas for this book, offering to publish the book, and encouraging me to get it done. Their gentle prodding and wise guidance assured its successful completion. Heather Garnos Mitchener, the editorial manager at New Harbinger, provided immeasurable help in editing the initial manuscript and turning it into a readable and hopefully enjoyable book. Carole Honeychurch, my copyeditor, deserves credit for making this manuscipt more readable. I also thank Michele Waters, the book design and production manager and Amy Shoup, the art director. Working with New Harbinger Publications was a very positive, enjoyable, and "pain-free" experience.

For this second edition, I wish to thank Mark Tracten of Crown House Publishing Company for seeing the value in publishing a second edition of the book after the first edition went out of print. His help and that of David and Karen Bowman of Crown House have been invaluable and very much appreciated. Re-publishing this book and the accompanying CD as been a pleasure with their help.

Last but not least, I thank my wife Andrea, my mother Cecile, and my late father Joe, for standing by me all these years, and my two daughters, Marisa and Allison, for tolerating a dad who could not always give them all of the attention they so much deserve. The love I give and receive from these dear individuals continues to make my persistent pain more tolerable.

*Bruce N. Eimer, Ph.D.*

*November 19, 2007*

# Foreword

Few people seem to realize that hypnotic healing is just the well-directed use of a common ability of humans. Anyone who can daydream can do hypnosis. Professor Ernest Hilgard's simple definition of hypnosis is "believed-in imagination." The two obstacles are in overcoming the disbelief and imagining (dreaming) the right goal. As the song in the musical South Pacific says, "If you don't have a dream, how're you going to make your dream come true?"

This book has much to offer the person with persistent pain who is willing to take the time and maintain the discipline to complete the exercises in each chapter. Pain comes without effort, and it's natural to just wish it would go away without effort. The nice thing is that when the time comes to induce trance, the change does take place without effort.

After describing hypnosis as we presently understand it and summarizing the story of his own pain, Dr. Eimer goes to the questions that need to be answered for a satisfactory understanding of pain and the coping style of the person who has that pain. Then there are choices offered about how to practice self-induction of trance and how to give the right **Self-suggestion.** I think it is particularly important to study chapter 8, which focuses on identifying subconscious, negative ideas and meanings that have outlived their usefulness.

A person with chronic pain can hardly avoid reflecting on its meaning and then imagining (daydreaming) other outcomes ("If only . . ."). Negative feelings of fear, anger, guilt, pain, and so on can be interchanged, so that pain will increase any fear that was already there, and guilt will increase the pain. The opposites of these negative feelings—courage, love, innocence, and comfort—are the daydreams that translate into relief. The word "pain" is derived from the Latin *poena*, meaning "punishment." Poena also gives us words like penalty and penitentiary. When guilt is an issue, there comes a time when one has been punished enough. The need then is to forgive oneself. When it's anger, you may need to forgive another, and if we are angry at God, we must forgive Him, too.

Bruce Eimer's search for relief from the pain of his own physical illness has led him to research and practice the self-hypnotic skills that have helped keep him from being an invalid. Pure pain without a psychic overlay is generally quite tolerable and is often of value in limiting overexertion. He has condensed this research into a book that is a summary of the best ways to understand the negative meaning an individual assigns to his/her pain, and how to change it with "believed-in imagination."

*—Dabney M. Ewin, M.D., FACS, ABMH Clinical Professor of Surgery and Psychiatry, Tulane University Medical School. Clinical Professor of Psychiatry, Louisiana State University Medical School. Past President, American Society of Clinical Hypnosis (ASCH)*

# Author's Foreword to the Second Edition

Since the publication of the first edition of this book, very little has changed in so far as the application of psychological and hypnotic techniques in the management of chronic pain and persistent pain syndromes. Few doctors and therapists have intensive training in this area. Many practitioners and patients remain skeptical of the value of hypnosis, self-hypnosis training and psychological techniques for relieving persistent pain and suffering. People generally turn first to drug interventions and medical/surgical procedures as these are what are reimbursed by health insurance companies.

Nevertheless, when all else has failed, many people who continue to suffer from persistent pain that has not responded to the gamut of medical treatments turn to alternative treatments such as acupuncture, hypnosis, imagery, psychotherapy, therapeutic touch, massage therapies, energy therapies, herbal remedies, etc.

I wrote this book to fill a gap in the self-help literature by providing a guide to using hypnosis, self-hypnosis and imagery techniques for managing chronic pain. I have used all of the techniques described in these pages in my practice with patients. Clearly, not all techniques work for everyone, but almost always I have found that there is a hypnotic technique for everyone or someone. In clinical practice, we assess the patient and explore which techniques have the greatest efficacy. The good thing is that, with psychological and hypnotic therapies, there is no significant downside issue of risks of negative side effects as there frequently are with drugs and surgery.

As the reader of this book, you will have the opportunity of exploring a wide range of hypnotic and self-hypnosis techniques for helping you to improve your ability to cope with and manage discomfort so that you can live more comfortably.  It is my suggestion that you read the entire book. However, how you go through it is your choice.

You may wish to read it cover to cover first and then go back to specific sections, or you may wish to read certain sections that appear to have the most relevance to yourself at this point in time.  However you choose to go through the material in this book is fine, and I am confident that you will find a way of doing so that will work for you.

I myself, being a person with chronic pain, also use many of the techniques in this book to maintain and promote greater physical and emotional comfort for myself.  In fact, I have been doing so for quite some time.  The techniques have been presented so that you can work with the exercises on your own, or with a knowledgeable therapist or coach, if one is available to you.

Of course, please understand that the material in this book is presented for educational purposes only, as it is impossible and unethical to diagnose or treat physical illnesses or mental, emotional or psychological disorders through a book!

Please be advised that any new unexplained pain, or change in your pain symptoms should be reported to a licensed medical physician.  It is irresponsible to attempt to mask pain symptoms that could be a signal of a medical condition that needs to be treated.  Remember that pain is a signal that something is wrong that needs to be addressed.  When everything medical has been done that should be done and can be done, then, it is time to explore psychological methods of coping.

This does not mean that you should not use good psychological coping tools in the acute phases of a painful condition.  I am saying that the first thing to do is to get proper medical treatment.  However, unfortunately, often medical treatments can only do so much, and you might be left to live with bothersome symptoms, or be forced to make hard choices.  This is when many of the techniques described in this book can really be helpful. Knowledge is power, and this book will impart knowledge to empower you.

Ultimately, we all must help ourselves.  Self-help requires knowledge, timely and accurate information, and a positive attitude.  These all figure into the process of developing the skills that are necessary for effective coping.

In this second edition of this book, we have added an additional component.  This is a 45 minute audio hypnosis CD.   This CD contains information about chronic pain and hypnosis, a hypnosis and relaxation induction, and a series of suggestions and exercises for improved coping with and management of ongoing pain. It is narrated by me, in my own hypnotic voice.

It goes without saying that this audio CD should only be listened to when you are in a safe and secure place where and when you can ignore outside distractions and turn your mental focus inward.

NEVER listen to this accompanying hypnosis CD while driving a motor vehicle or whenever your attention must be externally focused. To do so is irresponsible, and YOU are responsible for your own behavior.

This hypnotic pain relief audio CD features me leading the listener through a series of mindful exercises that teach gentle and safe ways to manage and relieve chronic pain. By listening to this CD, you will learn how to utilize the powers of your mind to gain greater control over your body through your mind, so that you can find your way to greater comfort.

While this CD was added as an accompaniment to this second edition of this self-help book, it stands on its own and can be used without the book. This CD uses Hypnosis to gently guide you into a state of relaxed concentration, awareness and inward focus. It teaches you the listener how to use Self-hypnosis as a coping skill for controlling chronic pain. The informative and pleasant suggestions on the CD are easy to follow, and the soothing and relaxing background music helps to further your experience of relaxation and comfort.

This Hypnosis CD is meant to be listened as often as you like in a safe environment when attention to external tasks is not required. It is designed to expand and improve your ability to control and cope with pain and diminish suffering with repeated listenings to the CD over a period of days. Each time you listen you reinforce your developing pain coping skills. Remember the old adage—practice makes perfect. Well, in this instance, practice makes better.

The CD specifically covers:

- What Hypnosis is

- Pain perception and Hypnosis

- Entering a relaxing state of Self-hypnosis

- Rating and lowering discomfort

- Pain relief and comfort imagery exercises

- Healing imagery

- Therapeutic touch and energy healing

- Comfort transfer techniques

- Instant stress control

The hypnotic and relaxation techniques on the CD are all described in detail in print in this book. So, please continue reading, listen to the CD at any point when you feel like doing so and it is appropriate to do so, and start getting more comfortable. I wish you peace and comfort and healing.

**Bruce N. Eimer, Ph.D.**

**September 18, 2007**

# Preface

*There is a mountain of hogwash written about patients inventing their pains . . . The patient's mood and attitude don't create pain, though the moods and attitudes of those around a patient well may be influential . . . The way we deal with pain is an expression of individuality.*

**—Patrick D. Wall**

Hypnosis for pain management is not a newly invented therapy or clinical application, but in fact has been employed with great success for more than two centuries (Gravitz 1988; Hilgard and Hilgard 1994). The use of hypnosis as a tool for relieving pain is not experimental—it is in fact tried, true, and proven. In this book, I'll focus on *your* role in being your own healer and your own subject or client. Therefore, in these pages, we shall be talking about ways to improve your relationship with yourself. All clinical applications of hypnosis recognized as valid by the experts highlight the important role of the relationship between the hypnosis practitioner and the client.

In this book, you will learn how to use self-hypnosis to relieve your pain. And in doing so, you will learn how to be your own hypnosis practitioner and a good client.

## ◎ How Is This Book Different?

If you have chronic pain, finding a health-care professional who can effectively treat you and help you find relief can be a very difficult and frustrating problem. Few physicians or other health-care professionals receive formal training in pain management. As a result, many health professionals reach a certain frustration level when they are presented with the problems of a patient with chronic pain, and as a result, they tend to shy away from treating such people. Yet there are quite a few excellent and readily available textbooks on pain management in the fields of medicine, nursing, and psychology that have been specifically written for health professionals. There have also been more than a few good books published on clinical hypnosis for health-care professionals that address the clinical management of pain.

Though it can be easily used by anyone, *Hypnotize Yourself Out of Pain Now!* is not written primarily for health professionals. It is for lay persons who have chronic pain and was written by a professional clinical psychologist who has chronic pain himself. So, you know the book is meant specifically for you, but now you may be wondering how can it help lay readers like you reduce their pain by using self-hypnosis. How is it possible for the lay person to be able to achieve this from a book? There are several answers.

This book makes it possible for people in pain to gain effective results in pain reduction through self-hypnosis because it first guides the reader in evaluating his or her pain, coping strategies, and hypnotic responsiveness. Then it gives the reader the choice of a number of methods for inducing self-hypnosis (meaning entering and enjoying the hypnotic trance state). Because you can choose the right self-hypnosis method for you, the method you choose will work.

This book helps you build confidence in your ability to use self-hypnosis to cope with and relieve pain thereby reducing the feelings of being helpless and trapped that so often come with persistent pain. As you read on, you will realize that you have choices, and that you can make a choice by exploring the methods and strategies that I describe in this book. No other book that I know of (either for professional clinicians or lay persons) does this in the area of using self-hypnosis for pain management.

When you've had pain that hasn't responded to treatment for a long time, it's natural to become disillusioned and expect nothing to work—let alone anything you read in a book. What this book does is provide a fresh look at the problem of managing persistent, physical pain using the tool of self-hypnosis, and this new approach comes from an experienced hypnosis clinician and clinical psychologist who is a pain sufferer himself (me!).

I wrote this book for anyone who has chronic pain and wants to get more relief and gain more control without drugs. It assumes no prior training in mental-health sciences, hypnosis, or psychotherapy, nor does it assume any prior experience working with a clinical hypnosis practitioner or psychotherapist.

## ◎ The Scope of the Problem

More than ninety million people in the United States today have some form of chronic pain. For many, the pain is persistent and severe enough to cause significant disability. In fact, chronic pain is the leading cause of disability in this country. When pain resulting from injury, disease, or physical impairment causes significant disability, it often brings untold suffering. "Pain" refers to the physical sensations of discomfort. "Suffering" refers to the experience of emotional distress and may include feelings of anxiety, fear, depression, grief, and anger. Suffering makes physical pain worse. While pain may be an unavoidable consequence of injury, disease, or physical impairment, suffering is not necessary. Pain may be mandatory, but suffering is optional.

## ◎ What This Book Will Give You

This book is the first published guide devoted entirely to teaching effective self-help techniques for hypnotizing yourself out of both pain and suffering. It will teach you how to evaluate and assess your own pain and how to use a variety of cognitive and self-hypnotic coping strategies to relieve it.

In the chapters that follow, you will learn self-hypnotic techniques for:

» "Reframing" and "decatastrophizing" your problems;

» Distracting yourself from unnecessary pain;

» Taking control of your life and directing your own behavior;

» Using deep relaxation as a coping tool;

» Positively transforming pain sensations so that they are less uncomfortable and bothersome;

» Dissociating and disconnecting from the pain;

» Uncovering and resolving hidden conflicts that make pain worse.

You will also learn a philosophy and practical, psychological pain-management strategies for building pain tolerance and inoculating yourself against unnecessary pain, stress, and suffering. I have endeavored to provide plenty of realistic and useful advice for readers who have tried everything else with little prior success. As a clinical psychologist who has treated hundreds of people with various chronic-pain syndromes over the years, I'm familiar with being considered a "court of last resort." I have helped hundreds of people who felt that they were in a sinking boat, individuals who had lost hope and felt ready to throw in the towel (or the oars) and give up.

Being that I am also a person with chronic pain due to a permanent injury, physical impairment, and a progressive disease, I myself have been through the gamut of treatments. I have experienced the frustrations of going from one health-care professional to the next with the hope of finding pain relief, only to be disappointed in the end.

One of the things that I have discovered as a result of my personal and professional experiences is that every person must ultimately take responsibility for his or her own behavior, feelings, thoughts, and experience. Pain is a behavior, a feeling, a thought, and an experience. Taking responsibility for how you cope with your pain constitutes a conscious choice. It is your choice—it's up to you how you handle it. Nobody but you can cope with your pain.

Self-hypnosis is one of the best nondrug tools we have for coping with persistent pain. So, if you're interested in exploring one more avenue for managing and relieving your pain and suffering, then this book is for you. *Hypnotize Yourself Out of Pain Now!* will teach you how to effectively use self-hypnosis for pain control. It is meant to be read and used. It contains useful information, ideas, concepts, stories, and practical exercises. If the ideas in my book appeal to you, then you will want to keep it handy and refer to it often.

## ◎ Please Keep in Mind . . .

To state the usual, necessary cautions, qualifications, and reminders, the information provided in this book does *not* constitute medical advice or treatment. That simply can't be provided by reading a book. Furthermore, this book is *not* a substitute for appropriate and necessary medical attention, advice, and care, or individual consultation with qualified, licensed health-care and medical professionals. Each individual's health concerns should be evaluated by a qualified, licensed health-care professional.

However, this book *is* meant for self-application, and therefore, it is user-friendly. Some readers may be able to use the practical information contained in this book on their own, while others may benefit from using this book in collaboration with a qualified health-care provider. In addition, it should serve as a useful tool for health-care professionals who work with people who have chronic pain. Persons seeking relief from their pain, and health-care professionals, should find answers to some of their questions within these pages, as well as a clearer understanding of chronic pain and its management.

## *Your Responsibility*

You are responsible for taking complete charge of your own emotional and physical well-being. Neither I nor anyone else can assume that responsibility for you. In order to benefit from this book, it's necessary that you understand and accept these facts. If you do not agree, it is pointless to read further.

You are in charge of you, whether you choose to seek help or not. When you do seek help, you should not think that you are resigning or surrendering your responsibility for your own choices, actions, and experience. Experiencing hypnosis under the care of a qualified, licensed health professional and hypnosis practitioner does not take away your control over your own experience or your responsibility to accept and exercise that control. If anything, it reinforces and strengthens your control and responsibility. The same conditions apply in learning to use self-hypnosis, as you will, in this book.

## **Whom This Book Is For**

I've written this for people with chronic pain who have not responded well enough to previous medical treatment. In these pages, I provide information, facts, exercises, and strategies to help you learn how to use self-hypnosis as a self-help tool for pain relief, and also to help you learn some useful "lessons" from your chronic pain. This book will serve as a useful adjunct to proper medical treatment. It will empower you in taking responsibility for your own choices, your own health and well-being, and taking charge of your own experience.

Ultimately, all of us who suffer from chronic pain must rely on our own resources. Medical doctors and other health professionals cannot cure us. Medicines and surgeries are only effective up to a point and usually have unavoidable, undesirable, side effects.

## The Issue of Side Effects

Most pharmaceutical medicines have side effects because they work by modifying one or more biochemical reactions or systems in the body. However, everything is related to everything else in your body. The body's systems work together synergistically, that is, in concert with one another. When a drug modifies one system, it also has effects on other, related systems. So, a drug may be effective in stopping or modifying one biochemical reaction, and thus halting a symptom. However, this may cause another biochemical reaction, which may then result in another symptom or group of symptoms (side effects).

In addition, with many chronic conditions such as chronic pain, most medicines are only effective up to a point in alleviating or controlling the symptoms of the underlying disease. In prescribing any medication, most physicians weigh the medication's potential benefits against the risks of side effects and the magnitude of the medication's most common side effects.

One of the benefits of using hypnosis to control pain is that there is no risk of negative side effects. Self-hypnosis is not like a pharmaceutical drug, which is an external agent that is ingested or injected and modifies biochemical and physiological processes. Self-hypnosis is an internal or inner method for communicating with the unconscious or subconscious mind, which is the part of the mind that controls all of the biochemical and physiological processes that keep us alive.

Because self-hypnosis is an inner method of self-communication, it is safe; the unconscious mind will simply not accept suggestions that are consciously or subconsciously deemed harmful or unacceptable to you. So, there is only a potential upside and no downside to using self-hypnosis to control and relieve persistent pain and discomfort.

Most people who have chronic, persistent pain are willing to try any reasonable treatment method if there is a chance that it can help them obtain pain relief and if the potential risks posed are not too great. Therefore, you really have nothing to lose and a lot of benefit to gain when you give self-hypnosis and the methods explained in this book a chance. But you should still continue to follow your medical doctors' advice as long as you continue to have faith in your doctors.

## ◎ A Most Important Qualification

Do not consider any of the methods discussed or explained in this book as substitutes for appropriate medical evaluation, treatment, and care. None of them are. This book is intended to inform and educate and also provide you with new choices for coping more comfortably and effectively with your pain. Some of the techniques described may also serve as adjunctive methods to complement your ongoing medical care. If you lose faith in your current care providers, find new ones. Share this book with your health-care providers. You may wish to tell some of them that you are reading this book and intend to practice the exercises in it. When you begin to use some of the methods you've learned from it, you may wish to share some of these methods with your health-care providers.

Reading this book will change the way you think about your persistent pain. I intend to equip you with the knowledge and skills that will enable you to better manage your pain and the "emotional overlay" accompanying it. The information, skills, and strategies that I will describe have been field tested by an experienced clinician who copes daily with chronic pain himself (that would be me).

I will also help you to remember what helpful things you've done in the past that you may have forgotten about. So, I will remind you about things you already know how to do and provide you with guidance on how to utilize these things in conjunction with the new things I will teach you. The famous psychiatrist and medical hypnosis pioneer Milton H. Erickson used to say that people already know how to forget about pain.

## ◎ My Story

When I first became injured in a major car accident in 1993, I began to learn firsthand what so many of my patients over the years had been going through. From my first visit to the emergency room immediately after the accident, I began to experience how alone we really are when we have severe pain. From that point on, health-care professionals, insurance companies, and some friends and family questioned if I really was in that much pain, and if so, how that could be. After all, some said, I looked a lot better than my totalled Jeep Grand Cherokee did, and I survived!

Quite to the contrary—I was in pain *because* I survived! As I shall discuss later, the pain served an all-important signalling function—to alert my unconscious that I did survive, and that I was alive.

Even when I was writhing in agony on the floor in my house before I was admitted to the hospital to await back surgery, some people questioned and wondered how I could be in that much pain. Here again, the overwhelming pain was serving an all important signalling function. It was telling me that I needed to have a surgical intervention to relieve the spinal vertebral disks' pressure and consequent damage to the nerves in my low back and leg.

I learned that pain is a very personal experience. No one but you can feel or even understand your pain. It also makes it worse when you feel that you have to justify your inability to perform your previous duties because the pain interferes so much. It just makes the pain worse when you feel that you must prove that you have pain. The pain is there for a reason. It is a reminder that life must be conducted differently. So I learned quite rapidly that I was better off not trying to convince others of what I was going through. They couldn't possibly understand anyhow. That was one lesson I learned from my pain.

Ironically, for years as a practicing clinical psychologist, I had specialized in treating people who suffered from chronic pain. I felt that I had usually been empathic. In fact, I had chosen this specialty because I realized early on in my clinical psychology residency training that people with chronic pain constituted a large, underserved population. Helping people manage their persistent pain, I realized, would create a very necessary and important niche for my practice. After my motor-vehicle accident at the end of 1993, I was in almost constant pain myself and scared about my future. So I pledged to myself that, once I was able to, I would do anything within my power to help other chronic-pain sufferers cope with the changes persistent pain brings about. Writing this book is one way I have attempted to do this.

I learned firsthand that medicines, physical therapy, and surgery can only help so much. When you have a permanent injury and physical impairment that impedes your functioning, you must find a way to cope. You have to find your balance. Severe, persistent pain is limiting and disabling.

I realized that I had to come to accept my disability and learn ways to come to terms with it and cope with it. I no longer could do what I used to be able to do. The key was to find meaningful ways to assure a good quality of life for myself and still be productive and creative, to keep my mind stimulated. I needed to find new ways to continue to contribute to society and to my fellow humans in pain, balancing this with my own daily pain management and all of my roles and obligations.

Eventually I found that writing was a way to keep my brain from becoming stale. An active, bright, inquiring mind is a terrible thing to waste. One of the most important ways that I learned to cope with my persistent pain was to make sure I immersed myself in stimulating, interesting activities, at a pace and schedule I could personally handle.

I discovered that staying out of pain was a full-time job. I learned that the best way for me to cope was to avoid stressful situations and conflicts as much as possible. I realized the necessity of focusing on doing things that I find pleasurable and fulfilling, such as writing, reading, learning, and teaching, *at a pace that I can tolerate.*

I have learned to follow the Ten Commandments for Coping with Chronic Pain (Bassman and Wester 1997). The first letters of these commandments spell the acronym NO MORE PAIN (Oh, do I wish!), and include:

» **N**oticing where I am relatively comfortable;

» **O**ptimizing the control I do have;

» **M**otivating myself to engage in positive activities;

» **O**pening my mind to new possibilities and choices (being flexible as much as possible);

» **R**elaxing in some regular way (i.e., using self-hypnosis regularly);

» **E**valuating my time and priorities (recall that managing chronic pain can be a full-time job);

» **P**racticing self-hypnosis to gain some control over my pain and other symptoms;

» **A**voiding stressful and conflictual situations as much as possible;

» **I**ndividualizing my schedule and not being afraid to make "downtime" when the pain flares up;

» **N**egotiating support from others.

I learned that regular, mindful exercise and movement within my tolerance limits, changing my physical position on a frequent basis, minding my posture, and frequent stretching, helped me to maximize my comfort levels, and keep my pain tolerable. I also discovered that keeping my pain under control necessitated keeping an open mind, maintaining balance in my life by adopting a balanced philosophy, and using the tool of self-hypnosis regularly.

Later in this book, I will be telling you much more about coping strategies that enabled me to do this. That is what this book is mainly about: realistic coping strategies for getting comfortable and getting out of pain. This is not to say that if you have a significant physical injury and impairment you can rid yourself totally of all pain or return to your pre-injury level of functioning. That is unrealistic. What is realistic is the goal of keeping pain tolerable, finding as much comfort as you can, and being as functional as you can be. Unfortunately, these goals do not always jibe with the expectations of insurance companies, employers, doctors, family members, friends, and so on. But, ultimately, you have to answer only to yourself and God.

Different parties have different agendas. Unfortunately, people with chronic and persistent pain often find ourselves caught between the conflicting desires and needs of the people and institutions around us. We have our own need to escape from pain, and then we must also face our insurance companies' desire to get us off of disability and back to work, our family members' need to have the "old you" back, and doctors who want to have a compliant patient who responds positively to the particular treatment the doctor provides. There's also the legal system trying to prove or disprove permanent injury of reasonably certain causation, and our employers' need to get us back to work as soon as possible, or "off their back."

Conflict creates stress and that stress is experienced both consciously and subconsciously. Stress makes coping with persistent pain more difficult than it already is. This dynamic tends to make pain worse. Unfortunately, conflict is often an omnipresent companion of people with chronic, persistent pain. One of the jobs of the "pain psychologist" is to help the patient review and reframe the circumstances and events that have been causing or maintaining the patient's conscious and unconscious conflicts, helping the patient resolve those conflicts. A relatively conflict-free person with persistent pain is more empowered to cope with the pain and more likely to get out of pain.

The unconscious (or subconscious) part of your mind is aware of conflicts that you may be unaware of on a conscious level. The unconscious controls all of your automatic habits and all of the functions that keep you alive (such as blood pressure, heartbeat, heart rate, breathing, digestion, sleep-wake cycles, etc.), including pain. You need to be able to communicate with your unconscious mind to help alleviate persistent pain. Hypnosis is the most effective, nondrug tool we have for communicating with our unconscious mind.

This book presents my understandings and philosophy about pain coping using the tools of hypnosis and self-hypnosis. The ideas I share with you are derived from my years as a practicing clinical psychologist and my firsthand knowledge of pain.

I have had almost fourteen years now of learning to practice in my own life what I have taught patients and health professionals. Given my personal relationship with persistent pain, I discovered that I had to modify many ideas and techniques to make them more realistic and practical, and I also had to learn new ones that really work. In this book I share with you all that I have learned.

Everyone responds to pain in their own way. As you read this book, you will learn the best ways for you to manage your pain. You will be helped to make choices. Because *you* will choose the self-hypnosis methods and hypnotic coping strategies that feel right for you, they will work for you. As you begin this journey, recall the wise words of Dr. Patrick D. Wall (2000), one of the world's foremost pain researchers:

*"The way we deal with pain is an expression of [our] individuality . . . Any knowledge that brings patients into a clearer appreciation of their condition decreases their anxiety . . . The fear of pain is often worse than the pain."*

# Part One

## Learn About Your Pain and How You Cope

*Now Jabez was more honorable than his brothers, and his mother called his name Jabez [literally meaning he will cause pain], saying, "Because I bore him in pain." And Jabez called on the God of Israel saying, "Oh, that You would bless me indeed, and enlarge my territory, that Your hand would be with me, and that You would keep me from evil, that I may not cause pain!" So God granted him what he requested.*

**—Chronicles 4:9–10**

# ONE

# Understand the Puzzle of Pain

*Pain is a warning signal; when everything that CAN be done and should be done has been done, there is no reason for it to continue. . .*

**—Kay F. Thompson, D.D.S.**

*Hypnotize Yourself Out of Pain Now!* is about learning how to apply, and getting into the habit of applying, the appropriate counterstimulation and competing stimulation to subdue and tame your pain. As you will learn, this involves learning how to refocus your attention and your mental energies to become absorbed and engaged in comforting and pleasurable mental activities. It's all about mentally shifting out of a state of discomfort into a state of comfort.

We will be talking about numerous ways to do this. This will help you regain greater control over your pain, your symptoms, and your experience. You will be presented with choices. By making these choices, you will become more successful at taking charge of your own experience and learning how to choose better.

## ◎ Pain is an Energy Drain

Living life and coping with life's demands requires a replenishing supply of energy. The more energy you have and the easier it is for you to renew your energy supply, the stronger you're likely to feel. Living with unrelenting pain is a persistent drain on your physical and psychological energy supply. Persistent physical pain can feel like an angry force inside that just wants to keep punishing you. Being punished relentlessly can take a lot of the fight out of you.

Persistent pain saps your well-being and depletes your strength and resilience. Life is difficult and demanding enough as it is. Add the inescapable challenge of having to cope with continual or frequently recurring physical discomfort and the demands and difficulties that life brings can really feel overwhelming.

If you have chronic, persistent pain, this book is written with the goal of helping you discover ways to ease that pain so that life can once again be more pleasurable and enjoyable. Pleasure is the opposite of tension and pain. When you are enjoying yourself and feeling relaxed, you cannot be in pain or feel tense, pressured, or stressed at the same time. This is because the feeling states of pleasure and relaxation are the opposite of those other feeling states. So when you learn how to really relax and enjoy yourself, you will naturally feel more comfortable. You will be able to do this better and better as you learn and practice ways of Entering a Neutral, Joyful, Open, and Yes kind of mood. It is not unintentional that the first letters of each of these key words spell the acronym ENJOY.

This little book will teach you how to do this—and it's easier than you may think. Trust me. Now I know that at this point it may be hard to trust anyone who claims to be able to help you ease your pain. If you feel this way, you probably have been disappointed many times before. However, you really have nothing to lose by giving me a chance. Believe me, I do understand.

# ◎ A Definition of Pain

As a first step in being able to control something, especially a puzzling phenomenon such as pain that won't go away, it is often helpful to be able to define it or at least describe it in terms that make sense. Therefore, I think that we should start by defining pain. The definition that I use is one that enables me to help alleviate it using the psychological tool of self-hypnosis. This definition is an adaptation of one provided by Price (1999).

*Pain is an unpleasant bodily experience that feels like something in the body has been or is being damaged or destroyed, that feels like a threat to or interference with one's ongoing functionality and health, and that is associated with negative emotions such as fear, anxiety, anger, or depression.*

This definition acknowledges that pain contains several elements or components: 1. a bodily *sensation* with qualities like those experienced during or after tissue-damaging stimulation, 2. an experienced *threat* or *interference* with one's functionality associated with this sensation, and 3. an *emotional feeling* of unpleasantness or other negative emotions based on this experienced threat or interference.

So pain contains a *sensory* component and an *emotional* component. These two components are intertwined in the experience of pain. Yet one of the keys to relieving pain is to disentangle these two components, to separate the sensory or physical from the emotional or mental components of the experience.

All pain contains a physical or sensory component, and an emotional, mental, or psychological component. All pain is a very subjective, very individual, very personal experience. Nobody can feel your pain like you can, no matter how much it hurts or how well you describe it.

The definition of pain that I have adopted does not require you or anyone else to "objectively" demonstrate, as through CAT scans, or X rays, or MRI scans, or blood tests, actual or potential tissue damage. It does not require that an association even be made between the unpleasant sensation and actual tissue damage. However, it also does not eliminate the possibility that the pain is related to some sort of tissue damage. If there is such a relationship and the tissue damage can be arrested or repaired, then there is the possibility of pain relief. So, appropriate and competent medical and physical evaluation and treatment should always be undertaken.

What this definition of pain accomplishes is to place the most importance on the *felt experience* of the person in pain. If a person says that he or she is in pain, then he or she is in pain. This means that we must not ignore the psychological component of the pain experience when we focus on the physiological aspects.

Such a definition of pain allows for a balanced view. It does not overemphasize the importance of medical-physical factors at the expense of psychological ones. On the other hand, it does not compromise the importance of medical-physical factors and overemphasize psychological factors. Pain is neither all in one's head, nor all in one's body—it is contained and experienced in both places. The mind and the body both play an equally important role in initiating and perpetuating the experience of pain.

This is a great advantage because it opens the door to the employment of psychological methods of intervention such as hypnosis for the alleviation and management of pain. As David Spiegel, M.D., a noted Stanford University research psychiatrist and hypnosis researcher, has stated, "the strain in pain lies mainly in the brain." To say "lies *mainly* in the brain" may be a bit misleading, however, because it can be taken to mean that pain is mostly a psychological matter. Things just aren't that simple. However, the fact is that the negative experience of pain is perceived via the mental faculties of the mind. If something is wrong in the body tissue, that must not be ignored. However, if it cannot be corrected or completely repaired, it still can be accommodated and adjusted to. So, I would add further clarity to the puzzle of pain by stating that *to tame pain, we must use our brain.*

Just for the record, the formal definition of pain developed by the International Association for the Study of Pain (Merskey and Bogduk 1994, 210) states that *Pain is an unpleasant sensory and emotional experience associated with actual or potential tissue damage or described in terms of such damage.* This definition also highlights that pain is an unpleasant experience with both sensory and emotional aspects, and that it is associated with perceived damage to the body.

## ◎ Types of Pain

All pain is not the same. First of all, an important distinction that needs to be made is between acute and chronic pain. *Acute* pain is pain that is of recent origin. For example, the immediate pain you feel when you stub your toe or burn yourself is acute. The new pain from a recent injury is also considered acute. With appropriate medical care and treatment, acute pain is supposed to eventually subside. However, as anyone with persistent pain knows firsthand, pain doesn't always go away even when appropriate medical treatment is provided. When pain lasts beyond the point where it should have subsided or gone way, it may be considered *chronic.*

**Acute Pain.** Acute pain fulfills a necessary function—it keeps us from destroying ourselves. It serves as a highly useful signal that the body is in danger or under siege. It signals current or imminent harm to the tissues of the body. Without the capacity to feel pain, the world would be a much more dangerous place. For instance, you could burn yourself irreparably without even knowing it. You might not know in time that your collar was too tight, or that the zipper on your garment was pinching your skin, or that your finger was caught in the door. Obviously this is not a healthy way to go through life.

**Chronic Pain.** Chronic pain is another story. Chronic pain is persistent pain that often has outlived its usefulness. It's pain that has long since passed the time when it was necessary as a signal to alert you that there was something physically wrong in your body that needed to be tended to and corrected or escaped. It's pain that has not responded to appropriate medical or dental care and treatment, and the key word here is *appropriate*. Chronic pain is unrelenting and unremitting. It is often pain that is way out of proportion in its intensity and the disruption it causes to its functions or usefulness as a signal of harm or potential harm to the body.

Some health professionals and pain scientists consider pain to be chronic if it lasts for three or more months without getting significantly better. Some require at least six months. However, it is my opinion that these time requirements are somewhat artificial standards, and that they can become misleading and counterproductive. I believe that the key factor in defining chronic pain is that the pain has not responded to appropriate and competent treatments beyond the period of time during which one would expect the pain to be alleviated and the body healed.

**Types of Chronic Pain.** All chronic pain is not the same. There are many different types, with some of the more common ones including: recurrent headaches (such as those of the migraine, cluster, tension, or sinus variety); continuous facial and jaw pain often associated with a condition called temporo-mandibular joint syndrome (TMJ); persistent neck and/or shoulder pain; low-back pain; arm, wrist, and hand pain associated with carpal tunnel syndrome or thoracic outlet syndrome; the continual, intense burning pain and hypersensitivity of the skin, muscle, and nerves associated with conditions such as reflex sympathetic dystrophy (RSD) and post-herpetic neuralgia (PHN); the burning, shooting leg pain associated with sciatica caused by lumbar disk disease; the aching, stiffness and soreness associated with osteoarthritis and rheumatoid arthritis; the multitude of symptoms, associated with fibromyalgia; the persistent uncomfortably loud ringing or buzzing in the ears associated with tinnitus; the cramping, stabbing, jabbing, piercing, knifing, shooting, or squeezing pains associated with irritable bowel syndrome (IBS) as well as inflammatory bowel disease; and the intense cramping, pressing, jabbing, and soreness associated with persistent, unexplained pelvic pain.

**Pain May Be Mandatory, but Suffering Is Optional.** I've referred to this crucial statement earlier in the book, and I emphasize it here because of the essential idea it represents. That is, if we can find a way to subtract the emotional suffering element, what would be left would not likely hurt as much! Pure pain as a pure sensation, by itself, is not as persistently wrathful, punishing, or extremely bothersome as pure pain *plus* emotional suffering.

**The Puzzle of Pain.** Pain is both a puzzle and a study in contrasts. That is because it can be both our greatest friend and ally or our greatest antagonist. As a friend, acute pain and even, to a degree, chronic pain helps us survive. Acute pain is a signal or warning of current or potential or imminent harm to the body. But chronic pain untamed and uncontrolled can become a fierce enemy that makes life feel unbearable. However, chronic pain can also function as a friend. That is because, when there is underlying physical disease or injury, chronic pain can remind us of our limits. When heeded, it can warn us not to overdo it, to pace ourselves, and let us know what activities are unsuitable for us. If we ignore this warning, we can stretch too far and too fast past our limits and cause further injury to occur. The key point is that chronic pain can perform this signaling function without having to cause undue suffering. Maximum discomfort is not necessary. The pain may be able to signal you and serve its protective function without having to be that intense.

So pain, both acute and chronic, must be tamed and managed to remain our friend and ally. I shall be using the concepts and tools of hypnosis to teach you to tame your pain enough to again make it your friend. These concepts and tools will be explained to you in enough detail so that you will be able to benefit from trying them out and using them on your own.

As I shall explain later, hypnosis is probably the most powerful nonnarcotic tool we have to help people move from a state of discomfort to a neutral state or state of comfort. That is what I mean when I say that you can learn how to hypnotize yourself out of pain now. Comfort has a way of spreading and generalizing, just as discomfort and pain does. Once you get the comfort ball rolling, so to speak, it builds momentum and keeps rolling.

Self-hypnosis can serve as a very useful tool that you can learn to use to ease your chronic pain and manage and cope with it better. However, given all of the misconceptions and myths about hypnosis that abound, it is an underutilized tool. In chapter 3, I shall clarify these misguided notions so that nothing need stand in the way of your using this tool successfully. Amazingly, up until now, there has been no self-help book written for lay persons covering this topic in enough depth to help people with chronic pain. This book may just be the first!

Now, this book is no substitute for getting adequate medical attention and care. This bears repeating. Nobody should try to treat themselves. That would be foolhardy. It is essential that, before you seek to use the methods and techniques in this book to reduce your pain by yourself, you first seek appropriate and competent medical attention to evaluate and treat the source or cause of the pain.

Persistent pain demands an adequate medical workup *before* you start to rely on any psychological methods to mask, reduce, or cope with the pain. Not doing so would be like trying to ignore acute crushing pain in your chest radiating down your arm that could possibly be signaling a heart attack. To try to ignore or mask medically undiagnosed pain that could be signaling a correctable physical problem, or threat to the body's integrity, is very foolish.

The psychological and hypnotic methods discussed in this book can be useful once you know the source of the pain, or once you know that everything that can be done medically has been done. Some of the methods we shall discuss can also sometimes be useful in acute injury situations to keep you together psychologically until you can get adequate medical attention.

This book may also be used profitably if you are in therapy or counseling with a licensed counseling professional or psychotherapist, such as a clinical or counseling psychologist, clinical social worker, psychiatrist, pastoral counselor, psychiatric nurse, or mental-health counselor who uses hypnosis as a clinical tool. The ideas and exercises in this book can be worked through with the assistance of your psychotherapist or health professional.

However, this book is intended to be of help to you whether or not you are currently going for psychotherapy or counseling. It is just that, often, hypnosis has the most profound and lasting positive effects when it is experienced initially in a therapeutic situation. In such a situation, a licensed health professional would first help you to experience the hypnotic trance state. Then he or she would administer to you appropriately individualized and therapeutic hypnotic suggestions, including instructions for entering the hypnotic state by yourself. That means that he or she would teach you how to do self-hypnosis. In chapter 10, I will tell you how to select a qualified clinical hypnosis practitioner.

I shall be teaching you how to use self-hypnosis in this book. But first we will need to cover some important preparatory issues before you are ready to learn self-hypnosis for pain management. In chapter 2, I will help you to evaluate your pain, its effect on your life, and how you cope. In chapter 3, I will help you understand what hypnosis is and what it's not, and I will guide you in exploring your hypnotic and imagination abilities.

All of this information will help us to individualize your personal prescription for hypnotizing yourself out of pain in part 2 of the book. In part 2, you will be guided in choosing the right self-hypnosis induction methods and hypnotic coping strategies for you. Equipped with these powerful tools, you will be prepared to tame and manage your pain.

## ◎ The Physiology and Neurology of Pain

This section will summarize as simply as possible the medical understanding that we have to date of the physiology and neurology of pain. Gaining this understanding will help you to appreciate the key role that psychological methods such as hypnosis can play in helping you control and diminish your chronic pain and suffering. You may wish to read this section over as many times as you need to so that you will understand the main ideas.

**The Brain Is Like a Computer.** The human brain can be thought of as a computer. Like a computer, it contains the equivalent of a central processing unit (CPU) or motherboard. It can also be thought of as a central control room that contains a central switchboard or control panel. The spinal cord can be thought of as a bundle of telecommunication wires that transmit sensory messages in an electrochemical form to and from the brain.

The control panel or motherboard in your brain controls the transmission of pain and other sensory messages via the nerve fibers that run in tracts or bundles up and down your spinal cord. It also makes sense of the nerve signals that arrive after they have traveled up your spinal cord, and it sends messages and commands back down the spinal cord to those parts of the body involved.

Self-hypnosis can enable you to gain control over the "switches," or "chips," that control pain sensations in different parts of your body. These switches can be turned on or off mentally when you learn specific skills for doing so. You will learn these necessary skills later.

**Pain Amplification Syndrome.** Pain researchers such as Ronald Melzack, Patrick Wall (Melzack and Wall 1982; Wall 2000), and Donald Price (Price 1999) are learning how continued pain actually can cause the brain and central nervous system to become *hypersensitive* to pain signals and other, nonpain signals from sensory receptors in the body. They believe that persistent pain causes a kind of "neurological matrix," or vicious loop or cycle, to develop that keeps pain sensations going and going, so that the person in pain cannot get out of the loop. This can lead to the unfortunate emergence of what they call "pain amplification syndrome," wherein a system is established in the nervous system that amplifies even the smallest pain sensations.

One example of this is "phantom limb pain." Melzack and his associates have studied "phantom limb pain" (Melzack 1996) as one fascinating but unfortunate example of this phenomenon. This is a little-understood condition that affects some people who have had a limb amputated. Severe burning pain is felt in the area where the diseased or traumatized limb once was, but there are no longer any sensory nerve endings or receptors where the pain is felt because that portion of the limb is gone! So, if the nerves are gone, how can there be any pain?

According to Melzack, a neurological circuit or matrix somehow gets imprinted in the central nervous system. Apparently, nerve fiber tracts or bundles in the back of the spinal cord, where pain signals are normally transmitted, continue to fire in the absence of real sensory input from the severed limb. To complete the circle, the parts of the brain that interpret nerve signals as pain continue to interpret these false nerve signals and sensations as pain in the nonexistent limb. If the brains of people who have this condition are transforming false messages and sensations into very real pain perceptions, then we know that pain definitely is much more than just a simple sensation on a neurological level.

So, in this situation, the pain is really a memory that is experienced as very real, present pain. Is it all in the person's head? I don't think so. All in the person's central nervous system and autonomic nervous system (the part of the nervous system that controls physiological functions vital for survival)? I think partly. The pain amplification syndrome is also perpetuated in the muscles and soft tissues by muscle tension and spasm. For example, in chronic pain disorders such as fibromyalgia, myofascial pain syndrome, neuralgias, and reflex sympathetic dystrophy, the nervous system and muscular system are locked in a *neuro-muscular pain matrix* that amplifies or intensifies both painful and ordinarily nonpainful stimuli.

**Hypnosis Works in the Central Nervous System.** This is a definite "green light" to proceed with full confidence in the value of pain relief methods such as hypnosis. That's because hypnosis produces its analgesic (pain relieving) effects by altering a person's brain state, and the brain is the computer that controls the nervous system and the muscles. Hypnosis also *switches* on that branch of the autonomic nervous system that restores rest and relaxation while *switching off* the branch that pumps you up when there is a perceived threat to your well-being.

So relieving or taming chronic pain involves breaking up the vicious cycle in the central nervous system that produces pain amplification syndrome. In order to do so, it is necessary to somehow retrain your central nervous system to be less sensitive to pain signals. You will learn self-hypnosis methods for doing so later.

**Psychological Factors.** Psychological factors (such as thoughts, attitudes, beliefs, perceptions, emotions, behaviors, and habits) influence and regulate how your central nervous system processes pain sensations. They can cause your central nervous system to amplify pain sensations, or dampen them. Hypnosis and self-hypnosis are the best psychological tools we have available for altering our thoughts, attitudes, beliefs, emotions, behaviors, habits, perceptions, and experience.

**Chronic Pain Is a Serious Medical Problem.** Current research is beginning to prove scientifically that all types of chronic, persistent pain constitute serious medical problems (McCaffery and Pasero 1999). Unrelieved persistent pain causes physical and psychological stress due to the body's attempts to adjust to it. It can cause the heart to work harder and blood pressure to rise, as well as a host of other physical stress responses. Having to deal everyday with unrelieved chronic pain is likely to cause anxiety and depression, both of which worsen pain. This means that relieving chronic pain requires that this "emotional overlay" be addressed effectively.

In summary, people with chronic pain, rather than becoming desensitized, habituated, and less sensitive to pain as a result of having it around so much, actually tend to become *more* sensitive to pain. This appears to result from the central nervous system's attempts to adjust and adapt to the ongoing painful or noxious stimulation. Self-hypnosis can help you reverse or control this process.

# ◎ The Pain Gate Control Theory

Melzack and Wall (1965, 1982) have proposed the "Pain Gate Control Theory" that helps us understand how this pain amplification process can get started and imprinted in the central nervous system, and also, how this process gone awry may be stopped or remedied.

**Your Brain and Spinal Cord.** Nerve impulses are transmitted by bundles or tracts of specialized nerve fibers in your spinal cord from sensory receptors in your skin, muscles, and visceral organs to and from your brain. When nerve impulses reach your brain, they are processed and interpreted. Your brain then sends nerve signals down your spinal cord to instruct the appropriate parts of your body to respond to the original stimuli. If your brain interprets the signals it has processed as a threat or as pain, then the messages it sends back down to your peripheral nerves and muscles will direct them to act reflexively to protect you. Your first impulse will be to escape the perceived source of the pain or threat.

**The Pain Gate.** According to Melzack and Wall (1965, 1982), there exists a "pain gate" in the back of your spinal cord. This pain gate appears to control the transmission of nerve impulses to and from your brain by several types of specialized nerve fibers that run up and down your spinal cord. This pain gate is believed to be an actual neurological mechanism that can open or close the "nerve highway" in your spinal cord to the transmission of pain signals. So, when the gate is *closed*, nerve messages carrying pain signals are blocked. When it is *open*, pain signals travel unimpeded.

**Sub-Acute and Chronic Pain.** One type of pain-transmitting nerve fibers, called "C-fibers," is believed to open the pain gate by permitting pain sensations to travel up the spinal cord to the brain. The nerve signals that these C-fibers transmit are in the form of heat or cold sensations, mechanical sensations (like throbbing, aching, stretching, pressure, shearing, rubbing, squeezing, gnawing), and chemical sensations (such as penetrating, burning, cold, hypersensitivity, soreness, itchiness, tingling, numbing). The pain sensations associated with the nerve impulses transmitted by the C-fibers are typically spread out and poorly localized.

This type of pain is not the kind of pain that occurs immediately after an injury, but rather some time after. It's usually the kind of pain that continues after the acute phase of an injury has passed (termed "sub-acute pain"). It is also the kind of pain that doesn't respond to treatment and outlasts its usefulness as a messenger (termed "chronic pain").

C-fibers are relatively slow transmitters of nerve signals and pain sensations. This means that other, faster-transmitting nerve fibers can be stimulated to send nerve signals up the spinal cord to the pain registration center in the brain *before* nerve signals from the C-fibers reach the brain. In effect, this can serve to *block* the messages from the slower-transmitting C-fibers from ever registering in the brain's central computer. This is one way that the pain gate can be closed to chronic pain. So, think of the "C" in C-fibers as *chronic* or *closed*.

**Acute Pain Transmitters.** "A-fibers," which are a group of nerve fibers that conduct nerve messages very quickly, are responsible for transmitting acute pain signals up the spinal cord to the brain. This is the sharp, well-localized pain that one feels right after an injury or tissue damage has occurred. Think of the "A" in A-fibers as *acute* or *adaptive*.

That is why, if you have chronic pain and you sustain a new injury or additional tissue damage, the pain associated with the new injury is what gets your attention temporarily. It supersedes the type of chronic pain that has been there already. Of course this is advantageous to our survival and adaptive because it serves the function of notifying us that something new is going on that requires our immediate attention. This is also another way that the pain gate can be closed temporarily to chronic pain.

**The Fastest Transmitting Fibers of All.** There is a specialized type of A-fibers that send nerve impulses up to the brain the fastest of all. These special A-fibers transmit sensations of pressure, touch, and vibration. When you rub or massage an area of discomfort, for example, these are the fibers that fire. Their signals reach the brain first, before the messages from all of the other nerve fibers.

This is the neurological reason why rubbing or massaging an area of discomfort often provides temporary pain relief. The rubbing and massaging provide a form of competing counterstimulation, or *distraction* (to be discussed later in chapter 6 as a pain-coping strategy), that can block the painful stimulation from reaching and registering in the brain. This then is a third way that the pain gate can be closed temporarily to chronic pain.

**Transmitting Messages from the Brain.** There are still other types of A-fibers that, instead of sending nerve impulses up to the brain, send nerve messages from the brain down the spinal cord to activate peripheral nerves, which in turn activate muscle fibers. These nerve messages are responsible for causing muscle spasms, and muscle spasms can worsen pain.

Once again, these nerve fibers also serve an adaptive function because they are responsible, after an acute injury, for automatically causing your muscles to brace and guard so that they can support and protect the injured area. The problem is that when this muscle bracing and guarding continues for long periods and becomes habitual, it tends to cause muscle spasm and more pain.

## ◎ Closing the Pain Gate

The Gate Control Theory helps us understand how hypnosis can "close the gate" on pain. Hypnosis can direct attention away from pain sensations as well as transform your perception of the pain sensations. This can inhibit or slow the transmission of pain messages from the source of an injury or tissue damage to the brain.

At the most basic level, nonpainful stimulation of the peripheral nerves (like massage and rubbing) can stimulate the fastest A-fibers, which in turn can inhibit upward traveling pain impulses transmitted by the slower

A-fibers and the slowest C-fibers. Remember that all of these fibers interact with each other in the back of your spinal cord.

If pain sensations are not blocked or inhibited before they travel up the spinal column, other mechanisms can still influence the final outcome; that is, *how* pain is perceived, and *how much* pain is perceived. One such mechanism is the intensity of arousal of the sympathetic branch of the autonomic nervous system. It is activated automatically when you encounter stress or threat. When it is activated, you go into "fight, flight, or freeze" mode.

This has been called the "fight-flight response." The sympathetic nervous system causes the release of chemical neuro-transmitters such as adrenaline and other stress hormones such as cortisol that tend to pump up the activity of the nerve fibers that transmit pain messages to the brain.

Things that turn down or turn off the fight-flight response can also modulate or turn down pain, closing the pain gate. One such factor is relaxation. This is because relaxation is associated with the activation of the opposing branch of the autonomic nervous system, the branch that controls rest and restoration of body functions. It is called the *parasympathetic* branch of the autonomic nervous system.

A second pain-modulation factor that closes the pain gate is the stimulation of certain neurotransmitter pathways, specifically the ones that release and transmit the chemical neurotransmitters *serotonin* and *noradrenaline*. These internal chemicals dampen the upward transmission of pain impulses to the brain. They also inhibit the neural pathways that cause muscle spasm, which we know worsens pain.

It is because of this fact that certain antidepressant medications that make more serotonin and other neurotransmitters available help in controlling pain as well as depression. I am referring to the classes of drugs called serotonin re-uptake inhibitors (SRIs) and tricyclic antidepressants (TCAs). Some anti-anxiety medications also help in restoring the balance of helpful neurotransmitter chemicals.

A third pain-inhibitory mechanism that closes the pain gate is the stimulation of the body's production of internal opioid-like chemicals. These are called *endorphins* (meaning endogenous or internal morphine) and *enkephalins*. These neurotransmitter chemicals bond to the same opioid receptor sites in the central nervous system as do external opioid pain relievers that are ingested or injected, such as morphine, codeine, or methadone.

A fourth pain-inhibitory mechanism involves controlling and diminishing the negative emotional overlay associated with pain: a person's negative mood states, and negative thoughts, beliefs, and attitudes. Chronic pain associated with anxiety, depression, and anger hurts a lot more and causes a lot more suffering. That is because these uncomfortable emotions tend to be associated with the experience of helplessness, hopelessness, doom and gloom, and punishment.

# ◎ Pain Is a Complex Experience

The central concept in Melzack and Wall's Gate Control Theory is that pain is a complex experience that is mostly determined by what happens in the central nervous system as opposed to being determined solely by the stimulation of peripheral sensory nerves. Additionally, messages sent down the spinal cord by the brain itself are also believed to diminish pain perception. The way this is believed to work is to slow or inhibit the ascent of pain impulses up the spinal cord to the brain in the first place.

Chronic pain is at least partially maintained by an abnormal excitability of the nerve fibers that send pain messages up to the brain and a lack of effective mechanisms in the brain for dampening the transmission of these messages. As a result, a low-intensity painful, or even nonpainful, stimulus can actually elicit or aggravate pain. This is the pain amplification syndrome mentioned earlier.

This phenomenon and its resulting conditions are very responsive to the use of hypnosis when the person affected is positively responsive to hypnosis. Apparently, hypnosis somehow closes the pain gate in the central nervous system in a way that is not as of yet fully understood. Hypnosis works on multiple levels simultaneously. It influences a person's *cognitive* responses (their beliefs, attitudes, and thinking processes), *affective, emotional*, and *motivational* responses, and *sensory, perceptual*, and *motor* responses to address the complex problem of pain in an effectively complex way.

## Cognitive Factors

A person's beliefs, attitudes, expectations, and learning history influence how that person perceives and interprets pain, and that perception affects how the person experiences the pain. These *cognitive* or "thinking" factors activate the spinal cord's descending nerve pathways. The types of thoughts a person has and continues to think actually influence whether these descending pathways inhibit the ascent of pain messages up the spinal cord to the brain or stimulate their ascent. Positive thoughts tend to inhibit and negative thoughts tend to stimulate the ascent of pain messages.

## Three Dimensions of Pain

Melzack and Wall were the first pain scientists to classify the perception of pain into three basic dimensions or components. These are: the sensory dimension, the cognitive dimension, and the motivational-emotional dimension.

**The Sensory Dimension.** The *sensory* dimension is the lens or portal through which you discriminate the specific sensory qualities of your pain; that is, what the pain sensations feel like to you (for instance, sharp-dull, hot-cold, deep-shallow).

**The Cognitive Dimension.** The *cognitive* dimension is the gauge that you employ to evaluate your pain (considering it harmful or harmless, tolerable or unbearable, annoying or awful).

**The Motivational-Emotional Dimension.** The *motivational-emotional* dimension is what gives your pain meaning. It sets the emotional tone. For example, if your pain resulted from an injury intentionally inflicted by another person or from another person's negligence, then your pain's meaning is likely to be tied up with emotional factors such as rage, suffering, and the desire to extract retribution. On the other hand, if your pain is associated with a progressively worsening condition or disease, it will have a different meaning. Alternatively, if your pain is associated with having successfully gotten out of harm's way and surviving, it's likely to have a still different meaning.

The physician Henry Beecher (Beecher 1946) commented on this dimension after World War II. His thoughts were based on his observations of wounded American soldiers on the Anzio beachhead in Italy whose injuries sent them out of the battle zone. He noted that the wounded soldiers did not report as much pain as did civilians with similar injuries who were awaiting surgery in the United States. For the soldiers he observed, their injuries were their ticket home and out of the danger zone. Their pain was a conscious as well as unconscious reminder of this fact. Such was not the case for the civilians.

Your experience of pain is affected by the interaction of these three dimensions—sensory, cognitive, and motivational. Your mood states affect your perceptions of your pain's qualities and severity. Depressive, anxious, or angry mood states typically exacerbate or intensify chronic pain. These negative mood states are also associated with negative and dysfunctional thoughts, self-talk, beliefs, and behaviors. This is another reason why certain antidepressant and anti-anxiety drugs can help in relieving pain.

On the other hand, positive emotional states can ward pain off, or decrease its felt intensity. This would encompass mood states associated with pleasant emotional involvement, absorption in an activity, the drive to accomplish something considered worthwhile and meaningful, satisfaction in an accomplishment, dedication and devotion to another person or cause, and the feeling of gratitude.

In the heat of the game, the trained athlete ignores or doesn't notice their pain. The pain sensations are swept aside by the drive to outperform the competition and win. In between games in a series, the athlete's burning desire to perform at their best at the next event provides the motivation to consider the pain a distant second in level of concern and attention. It's not that the pain's signal is not heeded. It is just that the signal and the injury it heralds are considered part of the price that has to be paid to win. The pain signal is heeded with the goal of tending to the injury so that the athlete can stay in the game.

Of course, in most high-performance sports situations, the athlete views their pain as acute and temporary. There is usually an end in sight. While this is not the case with chronic pain, there is still something valuable to be learned from the professional athlete. The athlete's positive attitude and never-give-up spirit in the face of great physical pain associated with injury can be very inspiring (especially if the injured athlete is on your favorite team!). This highlights the fact that the meaning of pain is determined by, among other things, the context in which it is experienced.

## ◎ Solving the Puzzle of Pain

While we do not understand everything about the mechanisms of chronic pain, we do know about factors that can increase it and reduce it.

We know that "the strain in pain" is influenced by the brain. We know that hypnosis reduces the strain of pain by inhibiting the ascent of pain messages to the brain, or changing the way they are interpreted. However, before you can use hypnosis effectively to reduce your pain, you need to evaluate and understand your particular type of pain, and your responses to it.

# TWO

## Evaluate Your Pain and How You Cope

*Those who have trouble mastering pain usually have wrong ideas about the meaning of their pain, or attitudes about it that get in the way of overcoming it. In working with thousands of pain patients over the years, I noticed that those who are successful in coping with pain have certain attitudes in common.*

**—Richard A. Sternbach, Ph.D.**

The first step in hypnotizing yourself out of pain is to evaluate your pain. This will provide you with a basis for deciding what needs to be changed and what can be changed so that you can learn to cope better and feel more comfortable.

As I explained in chapter 1, pain has sensory, motivational-emotional, and cognitive-evaluative components. You need to understand these three separate but related components of your pain experience so that you can work with what you have to get better. To rephrase Dabney Ewin's wise statement that I quoted earlier, pain may be inevitable, but suffering is avoidable. Suffering is one part of the emotional component of the pain experience, and it can be avoided, averted, escaped, diminished, alleviated, and stayed.

## ◎ Chronic Pain: A Tough Adversary

I probably do not have to tell you that chronic pain is one tough adversary. Part of its toughness lies in its complexity. As time goes on, persistent pain tends to weave itself into the very fabric of your life, finding its way into all kinds of places where it's not welcome. Part of the struggle of coping with chronic pain is preventing the pain from taking over your life, or taking back control if it already has.

**Pain Is a Very Subjective Experience.** The same identical injury can produce a vast range of pain responses in different individuals. Just as no two people can experience pain in exactly the same way, no one can possibly know exactly what your pain feels like to you!

Pain is much more than an unpleasant physical sensation you experience solely in the present moment. Pain is a total physical and psychological experience. Everyone describes pain in their own unique way. Pain is a very subjective experience that is colored by a complex of factors in addition to the nature of your bodily injury and tissue damage.

These factors include your current situation, the implications of the pain for your life (personal, vocational, financial), other people's reactions to you and your condition, your personality and coping style, personal history, memories of the past, and plans and expectations for the future. Also included are your ideas about the meaning of your pain, and your attitudes about it.

**Before You Start the Process of Change.** Before you start the process of change and before you learn self-hypnosis, you need to evaluate these pertinent factors. Self-evaluation is the first phase of self-change. Once you know what these factors are, self-hypnosis can be an excellent tool for further exploring these factors and modifying them in a helpful way. Self-hypnosis, as I shall also explain, can enable you to start the process of change in the direction you desire and continue it.

So first you need to evaluate your pain and its effects on your life. Assessment and evaluation also constitute the first phase of treatment. You establish a baseline. Then, later on, you can evaluate your progress.

**First Get a Notebook.** For the following exercise and all of those that come after, I suggest that you get a notebook to write in. This will enable you to keep a permanent record of the information about yourself you have uncovered and what you have learned about hypnosis. Current research (Carpenter 2001) informs us that writing about stressful events and feelings actually reduces stress, especially if it involves analysis of the causes and effects of negative experiences and feelings, as we shall be doing here. Additionally, this research has revealed that keeping a written record of stressful experiences also reduces intrusive negative thoughts and feelings and improves working memory.

For each new exercise, start on a fresh page. At the top of the page, write down the date, the number and name of the exercise, and the page in this book the exercise appears on. This will enable you to keep track of your progress and refer back to the questions or instructions for each exercise at any time. I also suggest that you keep your notebook together with this book in a safe and secure place.

If you are currently working with a psychotherapist or clinical hypnosis practitioner, you may want to share the personal information you have recorded in your notebook with that person.

Remember, however, you do not need to be in therapy to benefit from this book. This book is written so that you can work through it, and benefit from the information and exercises on your own.

## Exercise 2.1: Evaluating Your Pain

The first step in evaluating your pain is to come up with a simple, easy-to-use "yardstick" or rating scale for measuring how much pain you're in, or the strength or intensity of your pain at any given moment. I have found that the simplest rating scale is a straightforward 0 to 10 scale, where 0 stands for "no discomfort or pain at all" and 10 stands for "the worst degree of discomfort," or "maximum intensity of pain you could imagine anyone ever having," or simply, "unbearable pain, the worst it's ever been."

**Self-Evaluation Questions.** The following questions give you words to say how it hurts. Your answers to these questions will help you later in developing effective self-suggestions to use with self-hypnosis. So, using your 0 to 10 rating scale, ask yourself the following questions now. Record your responses in your personal notebook. Keep in mind that how you rate your pain on this rating scale will naturally be different from how someone else rates their pain. That is all right. In fact, it's a good thing. You are not being forced to fit your way of thinking about the intensity or "badness" of your pain into anybody else's categories. What is most important is your experience, that is, how you feel!

1.   How would I rate the intensity of my pain or my degree of discomfort right now?

2.   What is the worst (most uncomfortable) that my pain gets?

3.   What is the least degree of discomfort I'm ever in?

You can use this pain-rating scale to gauge how you feel at different times of the day, after different activities, after treatments you might get, after you take any medication, and later, after you do your own self-hypnosis.

This method of rating or measuring your pain leads to the next three questions:

4.   Does the pain seem to be continuous, or always there, or does it seem to come and go? How long does the pain typically last?

5.   How much does the pain vary in intensity? Does it vary at all? A lot? Just a little?

6.   Do I know what seems to affect the degree of discomfort I feel? Certain activities? Certain times of day? The weather? What activities seem to make me feel more comfortable? More uncomfortable?

If your pain levels and experience vary, this is a good thing! When you're feeling more comfortable, you can imprint in your inner mind the feelings of greater comfort. You can borrow back a part of this memory whenever you feel less comfortable. You can remind yourself when you are less comfortable that the greater discomfort will pass. Remember that pain always changes. As Dabney Ewin says, "No pain lasts forever."

7.   How long have I had this pain? Do I know how the pain started?

Sometimes this is a hard question to answer on a conscious level. In chapter 8, I will teach you how to use self-hypnosis to obtain insights about such matters from your unconscious or inner mind.

8.   What have I done in terms of medical and/or alternative treatments? How about medical workups?

9.   How effective are the treatments I have tried for the pain? Rate each treatment's effectiveness from 0 to 100, where 0 stands for "not effective at all" and 100 stands for "so effective it gave me 100 percent relief."

You need not fall into the trap of "all or nothing" thinking about this. Accept shades of gray. There is a large territory between 0 and 100 percent. One therapy or self-help method may provide only 15 percent relief, but if you keep trying things, it all adds up to a new level of comfort.

10.    What do the doctors I've seen think is going on and causing the continued pain? Do I agree with them? What do I think is going on and causing the pain to persist?

Most likely, your physicians and health-care providers want you to get well. However, sometimes some of these professionals may make statements that, although well intended, are thoughtlessly worded. Think for a moment about the explanations your treating health professionals have given you about your pain. Were some of their words or statements uttered in exasperation? Did some of them explain things to you in highly technical medical language that you had difficulty understanding? Did those explanations ever lead you to wonder and construct grim pictures in your imagination?
It's important to get the facts about your particular condition and pain. Make sure to let your medical doctors know that you need them to explain things to you in terms that you can understand. That is an important part of their job. Remember Sergeant Friday from the TV show *Dragnet* whose famous line was, "Just the facts please, ma'am, just the facts."

11.    What medications am I taking now for the pain and otherwise? What have I taken in the past? How much pain relief do my medications give me?

The next few questions will help you describe your pain and any patterns you may observe. This information will be helpful later in developing and choosing self-suggestions for self-hypnosis.

12.    What does my pain feel like? How might I describe it to someone else?

13.    What color is my pain? What shape does it seem to have? What do I imagine it looks like? Does it travel, migrate, or radiate, or does it stay in one place? Is the discomfort on the outer surface of my body, or is it more deep or penetrating?

14.    What is my favorite color? What are my favorite feelings and sensations? What are my favorite activities? What are my favorite places?

15.    Is there any particular texture (rough, hard, bumpy) associated with the pain?

16.    In what ways does my pain vary in its qualities or characteristics? What different types of physical pain do I feel?

The information that comes up for you in answering these questions about your pain and later about your favorite feelings and activities will help you in selecting the most effective self-hypnotic coping strategies for relieving your pain. These strategies, as you will discover, focus on opposing qualities and characteristics to your pain. These opposing qualities are associated with greater comfort and relief.

Recognizing these opposing qualities will enable you to selectively recall pertinent pain relieving experiences stored in your memory when you need them in the future. In part 2, I will teach you how to utilize self-hypnosis to imprint such experiences and memories in your inner mind so that they automatically come to your mind when they can be helpful.

The next several questions are self-evaluation questions that require your being totally honest with yourself. They require that you answer to yourself and nobody else. They are key questions for evaluating how the pain affects you on an emotional and psychological level. Answering these questions will help you to gauge the degree of emotional overlay attached to your persistent pain, and your attitudes about the pain.

17.    How much am I bothered or distressed by the pain on a 0 to 10 scale where 0 stands for "not bothered at all" and 10 stands for "the most distress I could imagine anyone having"?

Notice that this question highlights the distinction between the intensity of the pain as a *sensation* and its *emotional* effects on you. The degree to which you're bothered by the pain gives some indication of how hard you may be willing to work to tame it and manage it better.

Dr. Frederick Evans (Evans 2001) recommends asking the following two questions:

18.    If suddenly I had no pain, how would my life be different?

Consider your response to question 18. Is it tinged with anger or impatience? Does it reflect the sense that it would make a world of difference or little difference at all if suddenly you had no pain? Do you think it would lead you to a major lifestyle change for the better? Is there a degree to which your pain saves you from having to resume doing something that you don't care to do?

19.   Do I want to feel better?

This question is a key one. As Dr. Evans (Evans 2001) suggests, I recommend that you ask yourself this question up to three times until you get from your self an "unequivocal YES!" Dr. Evans advises that you make special note of any answer that comes up for you other than a simple "yes." Listen to your self for any "yes, but" responses that come from within. Do you get a sincere "yes"? If you don't get a sincere "yes," ask your self why not. Ask yourself what it would mean if you did feel better, and what it would mean if you did not. You will derive the most benefit from this book when you are able to receive a sincere "yes" from your inner mind, pure and simple.

20.   If, as a result of reading this book and practicing the exercises in it, I was successful in reducing my pain by 25 percent would I be satisfied?

Naturally, you might prefer to be able to reduce your pain by a greater amount. However, if you can accept partial pain relief as a goal, you are more likely to achieve it. You may even get more than you initially expect, once you get the ball rolling. The point is to have realistic expectations and to be able to compromise. Aiming to obtain a little more comfort is more likely to pay off positively and sooner than aiming for total removal of the pain. A little more comfort is a lot better than no further comfort at all.

21.   Am I willing to work hard to get better?

The harder you are willing to work at it, the better your results are likely to be. Like with most things, you usually get back what you give or put in. Answering the following four questions will help you become more aware of how you feel about yourself.

22.   What do I like about myself? What don't I like about myself?

23.   What am I most proud of? What am I most ashamed of?

24.   When have I felt the most confident? The most accomplished? What has been my greatest failure? The worst mistake I ever made?

Your answers to the above questions can reveal inner psychological resources that you may be able to access in your efforts at taming your pain and getting better. Your answers may also reveal your vulnerabilities. Additionally, your answers may also reveal things that can motivate you to work hard to get better, as well as things you may want to avoid.

25.   What was the happiest time in my life? The saddest? When was I the most scared?

Your answers will clue you in to what have been your most pleasurable experiences, as well as some of the things that move you and affect you strongly—what you're motivated to seek out and approach and what you are strongly motivated to avoid or escape from.

Answering the following six questions will help you better understand your ideas about the meaning of your pain. At this point, you should be ready to answer this next set of self-evaluation questions.

26.   Knowing what I know now, what is my key problem? (If you feel that there are several, limit your answer to two key problems.) If you solve just one problem, the others may fall away naturally or become nonproblems.

27.   What does my key problem feel like? How might I describe it?

Again, your answer here provides useful information for designing self-hypnotic relief strategies that are geared to your individual needs.

28.   What does my key problem *stop* me from having, doing, or feeling? What does it lead me to have, think, do, or feel that I would rather not?

29.   What do I *want* most that I do *not* have now?

30.   What do I need to feel, do, and think in order to get what I want and to stop getting what I don't want?

31.   In order to get what I want, what am I willing to do differently from now on?

Your answers to questions 26 through 31 will help us set goals for change. Good goals are goals that are specific, realistic, honest, attainable, and easy to measure. Your answers will also help us develop appropriate suggestions that are geared to your individual needs.

# Exercise 2.2: The Pain Description Questionnaire

The Pain Description Questionnaire below is an adaptation of the well-known and widely used McGill Pain Questionnaire authored by Ronald Melzack (Melzack 1975). Dr. Melzack has given me permission to include some of his pain descriptors in my questionnaire. My questionnaire will help you describe your pain in plain language. It will enable you to pinpoint what your pain actually feels like by identifying the precise qualities your pain has. The questionnaire will give you words to say how and how much it hurts. We will use this information later in developing hypnotic and waking suggestions for pain relief based on opposing qualities that spell comfort. These opposing qualities will give you specific goals for your pain management geared to your individual needs.

## Instructions

You may wish to photocopy the questionnaire below to do this exercise, or you can use your notebook. If you choose to work with a photocopy, first put the date at the top of the questionnaire. Then, for each group of pain descriptors, first underline the one word that best describes or characterizes your pain. Then, use your 0 to 10 rating scale to rate how much of that quality or characteristic your pain usually has, or has on the average (where 0 means "none at all" and 10 means "the worst imaginable").

If none of the words in a group of descriptors characterize your pain, don't underline any word. Just put a 0 on the rating line for that group of words. Most people find themselves somewhere in between 0 and 10 for some or most of the items.

If you choose to use your notebook, turn to a blank page and put the date at the top. Then number each line on the page. For each group of pain descriptors, write down the one word that best describes your pain, and then place a number from 0 to 10 next to the word to indicate how much of that quality your pain usually has. Again, if none of the words in a group of descriptors characterize your pain or apply, just put a 0 next to that item number in your notebook.

For example, the first item asks you to consider how "intense," "strong," or "powerful" your pain usually is. Let's say you choose "intense", because it characterizes your pain the best out of that group of words. You then rate how intense your pain is on the average, or usually, from 0 to 10. You should do this for every group of descriptors.

**How [. . .] does your pain usually feel?**                                    **Your 0 to 10 rating?**

1.   Intense, strong, or powerful? _____

2.   Sore, tender, aching, or bruised? _____

3.   Sharp, stabbing, jabbing, piercing, knifing, or poking? _____

4.   Heavy, pressing, cramping, crushing, or burdening? _____

5.   Stiffening, tightening, or tensing? _____

6.   Deep or penetrating? _____

7.   Jolting, electric-like, lightning-like, or spiking? _____

8.   Shooting, blasting, bursting, or erupting? _____

9.   Radiating, surging, spreading, traveling, beaming, or flowing? _____

10.  Tearing, splitting, cutting, or ripping? _____

11.  Gnawing, chewing, biting, or pestering? _____

12.  Throbbing, pounding, beating, or hammering? _____

13.  Sensitizing, sensitive, raw, sore, irritating, or jumpy? _____

14.  Itchy, tingling, prickly, or stinging? _____

15.  Numbing, deadening, paralyzing, unfeeling, or dulling? _____

16.  Hot, warm, burning, on fire, or searing? _____

17.  Cold, freezing, or chilling? _____

18.  Persistent, nagging, stubborn, unyielding, or relentless? _____

19.  Constant, continuous, unremitting, interminable, or incessant? _____

20.  Unpredictable, mysterious, erratic, uncertain, or unforeseeable? _____

21.  Sickening, nauseating, or disgusting? _____

22.  Annoying, bothersome, troublesome, or disturbing? _____

23.  Tiring, fatiguing, or exhausting? _____

24.  Punishing, agonizing, tormenting, or torturing? _____

25.  Stressful, distressing, straining, overwhelming? _____

26.  Fearful, frightening, alarming, worrisome, or scary? _____

27.  Depressing, discouraging, disheartening, or demoralizing? _____

28.  Cruel, vicious, spiteful, malicious, or brutal? _____

29.  Unpleasant, upsetting, uncomfortable, hurting, or horrifying? _____

30.  Intolerable or unbearable? _____

## *Interpreting and Using Your Responses*

Note that descriptor groups 1 through 17 refer to pain's *sensory* qualities. These words may describe the physical character of the pain itself. Descriptor groups 18, 19, and 20 refer to the *temporal* qualities of pain; that is, how continual, persistent, and predictable the pain is. Descriptor groups 21 through 27 refer to your possible *emotional* reactions; that is, what the pain does to you. For example, "tiring, fatiguing, exhausting." Finally, descriptor groups 28, 29, and 30 refer to the degree of suffering the pain may cause; that is, how you *evaluate* the pain.

Your ratings for the emotional descriptors and the *evaluative* descriptors will help you get a sense of your degree of emotional upset associated with your pain. In chapters 5, 7, and 8 we'll cover strategies for reducing your emotional upset by changing your negative ideas about your pain and the meaning that you assign to it.

**Step One.** The first step in interpreting and preparing to use your responses is to note the pain descriptors that you rated at a 5 or higher.

Below is a list of *opposing* qualities for each pain descriptor group. These opposing qualities help you set goals for how you want to feel instead. For each pain descriptor you rated a 5 or higher, if you used your notebook, write next to your rating the opposing quality that has the most meaning for you. Feel free to add any personally meaningful opposing qualities that aren't listed. If you worked from a photocopy, also duplicate the following list and underline the most meaningful opposing qualities, as well as writing in any that you wish to add.

We will refer back to these opposing qualities later when we select pain-coping strategies and construct hypnotic self-suggestions. With self-hypnosis, you will be able to fix the appropriate opposing qualities in place in your inner or unconscious mind. Also, you will be able to select the appropriate opposing qualities to serve as your personal comfort cues, and to create effective post-hypnotic suggestions. More about this later. However, please keep in mind that these are some conditions that can cause such intense pain that no amount of positive imaging or mellowing seems to change the quality, character, or even intensity of the pain. I say this so that your expectations are appropriate and realistic.

If you have appropriate and realistic expectations, you will be able to deal with the pain more effectively, reduce how upset or distressed you get over it, and function better.

**Step Two.** The final step in interpreting and preparing to use your Pain Description Questionnaire results is to note your responses to certain key and especially problematic pain descriptor items. For example,

1. If you learned that you experience your pain as *sickening, nauseating,* or *disgusting,* one of your goals might be to learn to feel more *agreeable, neutral,* and *pleasant.*

Here are some others:

2. If you learned that you experience your pain as *punishing, agonizing, tormenting,* or *torturing,* you will benefit from learning how to use self-hypnosis to become more forgiving, peaceful, and loving.

3. If you find your pain or condition feels *intolerable* or *unbearable,* you will want to learn strategies for increasing your frustration tolerance, improving your ability to soothe yourself, and becoming emotionally and/or physically stronger.

4. If being *stressed out* and/or *overwhelmed* is your problem, you'll benefit by learning how you can use self-hypnosis to tap your inner resources so that you can make your experience feel more manageable, and so that you can begin to enjoy relaxing.

5. If being *depressed, discouraged, disheartened,* or *demoralized* is your problem, you'll benefit by learning how to use self-hypnotic techniques to psych yourself into experiencing what it feels like to be cheerful, at least a little bit happy, and yes, even grateful too!

6. If your problem is feeling that your condition is "totally" unpredictable or mysterious, you'll benefit by learning how to use your inner mind to uncover predictability in your symptoms and discover ways to achieve a greater sense of consistency and stability in your life so that you can feel better, more safe and secure, and become more functional.

Our next step, which will complete your self-evaluation process, is to evaluate how you cope.

## ◎ Evaluate How You Cope

To cope means to "handle," "endure," "deal with," "contend with," "manage," and/or "control." Chronic, persistent pain certainly is something to cope with, and when you are coping well, pain is less of an energy drain and you feel more comfortable. Therefore, my goal is to help you cope with your pain better.

## Pain Descriptors

1. Intense, strong or powerful
2. Sore, tender, aching, bruised
3. Sharp, stabbing, jabbing, piercing, knifing, poking
4. Heavy, pressing, cramping, crushing, burdening
5. Stiffening, tightening or tensing
6. Deep or penetrating
7. Jolting, electric-like, lightning-like, spiking
8. Shooting, blasting, bursting, erupting
9. Radiating, surging, spreading, travelling, beaming
10. Tearing, splitting, cutting, ripping
11. Gnawing, chewing, biting, pestering
12. Throbbing, pounding, defeating, beating, hammering
13. Sensitizing, sensitive, raw, sore, irritating, jumpy
14. Itchy, tingling, prickly, stinging
15. Numbing, deadening, paralyzing, unfeeling, dulling
16. Hot, warm, burning, on fire, searing
17. Cold, freezing, chilling
18. Persistent, nagging, stubborn, unyielding, relentless
19. Constant, continuous, unremitting, interminable, incessant
20. Unpredictable, mysterious, erratic, uncertain, unforeseeable
21. Sickening, nauseating, disgusting
22. Annoying, bothersome, troublesome, disturbing
23. Tiring, fatiguing, exhausting
24. Punishing, agonizing, tormenting, torturing
25. Stressful, distressing, straining, overwhelming
26. Fearful, frightening, alarming, worrisome, scary
27. Depressing, discouraging, disheartening, demoralizing
28. Cruel, vicious, spiteful, malicious, brutal
29. Unpleasant, upsetting, uncomfortable, hurting, horrifying
30. Intolerable, unbearable

## Opposing Qualities

Diluted, weak, subdued, powerless
Calloused, tough, insensitive
Dull, soothing, mellow, kind
Free, easy, light unimportant, supporting
Relaxing, limp, lenient, flexible, calm, loose
Shallow, superficial, simple, mild
Reassured, steady, soothing, calming
Contained, stable, safe
Flowing, absorbing, trickling, shrinking
Mending, joining, kind mild
Soothing, gentle, agreeable, delightful
Accepting, winning, yielding, quiet
Healing, indifferent, calm, pleased
Soothed, peaceful, contented, satisfied
Alert, sensitive, feeling, revived
Cool, comfortable, icy, calm, indifferent
Warm, passionate, in touch, comfortable
Flexible, forgiving, lenient, fair
Temporary, responsive, cooperative, brief
Predictable, consistent, stable, definite
Agreeable, neutral, attractive, pleasant
Neutral, pleasant, convenient, useful
Interested, refreshed, energized, easy
Forgiving, peaceful, comforting, loving
Kind, gentle, forgiving
Brave, comfortable, safe, calm, peaceful
Resourceful, strong, manageable, relaxed
Cheerful, happy, encouraged, grateful
Pleasing, healing, comforting, confident
Tolerable, mild, strong, soothing

The famous physician Dr. William Osler professed that it is much more important to know what sort of a patient has a disease than what sort of disease a patient has.

Understanding what your coping strategies are, what coping strategies are out there, and what strategies you favor will give you helpful insights about yourself. You will find these insights and this information useful later when I help you choose the right self-hypnosis method/s and hypnotic coping strategies for you.

# ◎ Coping Strategies

Psychologists have come up with different schemes for classifying people's coping strategies and this has helped us better understand the commonalities and differences among them. It also has enabled us to isolate certain key ingredients that appear to be associated with better coping and adjustment as well as with greater dysfunction and stress. I will briefly summarize what's important to be aware of here.

**Catastrophizing and Learned Helplessness.** The term "catastrophizing" means dwelling on, magnifying, and blowing up the negative aspects of a situation and expecting the worst. It means "snatching defeat out of the jaws of victory." Simply put, people who catastrophize think negatively, cope poorly, and feel no sense of mastery or self-efficacy. Do you catastrophize?

The term "learned helplessness" was coined by the University of Pennsylvania research psychologist Dr. Martin Seligman (Seligman 1975). It means feeling resigned to having no control over a bad situation, the way things will turn out, and believing that nothing you can do will make a difference, or change the situation. Do you ever feel this way?

Catastrophizing and learned helplessness lead to throwing in the towel, giving up, and getting depressed, which impede effective coping. These two stress-producing habits have been identified as the most significant predictors of poor coping and adjustment to persistent pain (Rosenstiel and Keefe 1983; Sullivan and D'Eon 1990). Reading this book and doing the exercises in it will help you to overcome these two traps.

## The Four A's of Pain Coping

Brown and Fromm (1987) have classified functional, psychologically oriented pain-coping strategies into four groups: avoidance, alleviation, alteration, and awareness. They have termed these the "Four A's."

**Avoidance.** To "avoid" means to avert, dodge, evade, escape, elude, or bypass. These are all things you want to do to escape the ferocity of persistent pain. "Avoidance" in this model refers to psychological coping strategies that direct your attention away from the discomfort. This strategy takes advantage of the fact that your conscious mind can only pay attention to a limited amount of information at one time. Since there are usually many things competing for your attention, you can distract yourself from discomfort by thinking about, or paying attention to, something else. Do you ever do this? Do you ever shift your focus of attention away from pain onto something else?

**Alleviation.** To "alleviate" means to ease, reduce, relieve, or soothe. "Alleviation" in this model refers to psychological coping strategies where you think about things that could make your discomfort diminish. For example, if you actually applied ice to an inflamed painful muscle, eventually that area would begin to feel numb and less uncomfortable. Now, knowing how ice feels on your skin, without actually applying the ice, you could simply imagine applying the ice. As you concentrate on how ice feels, your body will get the message, and that area will start to feel numb. Alleviation also encompasses the use of direct suggestions where you tell your body what you want it to start doing. Do you ever do this?

**Alteration.** To "alter" means to change, convert, transform, or modify from one thing into another. "Alteration" in this model refers to psychological coping strategies where you think about transforming sensations of discomfort into sensations that are more comfortable. For example, when you are floating, you cannot feel stiff or heavy. Similarly, if a body part feels uncomfortably hot, you can direct your imagination to make the heat dissipate and break up, helping you feel more comfortable. So, this is a way of substituting less bothersome sensations in place of pain sensations. Do you ever do this?

Alteration refers to changing the way you think about the pain. It could involve changing the way you interpret the pain's meaning, or imagining the pain as something else that is less uncomfortable. It could even involve imagining having the pain in another context or situation where you would be less concerned about it. Do you ever do this?

**Awareness.** To be "aware" means to be alert, attentive, and conscious. It means to observe or witness or watch what is going on with your full attention, without making any judgments about what is going on. Using awareness to cope with your pain means backing off and taking a passive attitude toward it, as opposed to trying actively to change what is happening. For example, if you make the pain sensations the focus of your awareness without making negative judgments, you are likely to notice changes in the intensity and character of the pain sensations. The pain's intensity may first seem to increase and then decrease. Pure awareness does require some practice, however. Do you ever do this?

## The Six D's of Pain Coping

I have been using another functional scheme for classifying psychological strategies for coping with pain (Eimer 2000a, 2000b; Eimer and Freeman 1998). I have labelled it the "Six D's." Each of the "D's" will be covered in detail in part 2 so that you can begin using them to get out of pain.

**Deep Relaxation.** This refers to the use of any of a number of methods for entering a deeply relaxed state or remembering and borrowing back the feeling of deep relaxation. When you're deeply relaxed, you cannot be in pain or feel distressed at the same time. The experience of deep relaxation is the opposite of these other feelings. Do you regularly use some form of deep relaxation to quiet your mind, calm your body, and release your tensions?

**Decatastrophizing.** De-escalating a tense situation by changing how you think about the pain and how you handle it is the essence of decatastrophizing. It enables you to put things into their proper perspective and transform adversity into advantage. Do you do this?

**Direction.** This one refers to taking responsibility for directing your own behavior. It involves taking charge of your life by employing a number of cognitive and behavioral coping strategies that help you gain control over your experience. Do you feel that you are in charge of your own behavior?

**Distraction.** This "D" involves refocusing your attention away from the pain. Do you do this?

**Distortion.** This involves employing your imagination to alter and transform your experience of pain sensations.  Do you ever do this?

**Dissociation.** This involves distancing, detaching, or disconnecting yourself from the pain so that you no longer feel attached to it. We shall be talking much more about this later. However, at this point, can you recall ever doing this?

Each of the six D's highlights an important aspect of using self-hypnosis for reducing pain. In the next chapter, you will learn about what hypnosis is and what it isn't.

# THREE

# Understand What Hypnosis Is and Isn't

*Whenever we become absorbed in what we are doing, we slip into hypnosis. Self-hypnosis results when you become absorbed in reading a book, in your work, in watching a motion picture or TV program, while listening to an interesting talk, even during some religious ceremonies. Any strong emotion may also produce hypnosis . . . Though these situations are not labeled hypnosis, that is just what they are.*

**—David B. Cheek and Leslie M. LeCron**

Myths and misconceptions about hypnosis abound. Much of what people think of as hypnosis is simply not true. The public, as well as many health professionals, have been misled about the true nature of hypnosis, the result of myths and distortions that have been promoted by movies, stage shows, and story books for purposes of entertainment. It's also the result of just plain misinformation.

## ◎ What Hypnosis Is Not

**Hypnosis Is Not Sleep.** When a person is in a hypnotic trance state, he or she is not sleeping. Therefore, a hypnotized person hears everything that is going on and is capable of responding to their surroundings appropriately. In fact, hypnosis has the unique quality of heightening or diminishing a person's sensory awareness, depending on what is needed at the time. The key phrase is "depending on what is needed at the time." Hypnosis can give a person more flexible control over his or her awareness, attention, and thinking processes.

**You Cannot Be Hypnotized Against Your Will.** No one can be hypnotized against their will. No one! You have to consciously want to be hypnotized to experience the altered state of consciousness we call hypnosis. If someone were to try to hypnotize you against your will, you simply wouldn't cooperate. Believe me. I have hypnotized thousands of patients. I have never been able to hypnotize any patient who was consciously resisting for any reason until I stopped, backed off, discussed the problem with the patient, and obtained the person's conscious consent to proceed and the patient's full cooperation and collaboration. If this was not possible, let's say because the patient had some ulterior motive, alternative agenda, or just didn't want to be in my office, we got nowhere.

In such cases, I level with the patient and make it clear that using hypnosis and doing effective psychotherapy is not a one-sided thing. It is a collaborative relationship that both the patient and the therapist have to want to enter into together for really valid reasons. In other cases, when I have detected unconscious resistance by the patient to cooperating with me, I also stop what I am doing, back off, and confront the patient so that we can discuss and explore in a waking state what is going on.

**Hypnosis Is Not about Swinging Pocket Watches.** Swinging pocket watches, pendulums, and crystal balls are the stuff of movies and story books. There is nothing special about a swinging pocket watch or crystal ball for the purpose of inducing hypnosis. These things can be employed as a visual fixation object (something to fix your attention to), but so can many other small objects. If a swinging, shiny pocket watch is used as a prop or aid to induce hypnosis, its purpose is to focus the subject's attention. Fixing your visual attention on any nearby interesting object can serve the same purpose.

**Hypnotized Individuals Cannot Not Wake Up.** Hypnotized individuals cannot not wake up because they were never asleep in the first place! If you do fall asleep while you are in hypnosis, then you are no longer in hypnosis; you are sleeping. When you wake up, you'll probably feel more refreshed, alert, and relaxed than you did before you fell asleep. An important question related to this myth that I would like you to consider now is the following: How often do you worry about not waking up when you take a nap or go to bed at night?

If you worry about this often, it has nothing to do with hypnosis. It is a fear. In fact, if your worries about this are severe, frequent, and interfere significantly with your life, you could have a specific phobia. Phobias can be effectively treated by a qualified mental-health professional. If a fear or phobia is very frequent, very severe, and impairs your functioning, it should be treated.

**Hypnotized Individuals Do Not Become Zombies.** A hypnotized individual is not paralyzed, incapable of taking care of him or herself, or incapable of refusing to carry out the hypnotist's suggestions or commands. The will of the person being hypnotized does not become subordinate to the will of the hypnotist. In hypnosis, you do not lose your decision-making capabilities.

You cannot be made to accept suggestions that are not acceptable to you. No hypnotist can make you do anything, experience anything, or change anything against your will. Some people call and ask if I can "make them" stop smoking. My answer, of course, is "No." I tell them that, if they are ready, I can use hypnosis to help them stop smoking more easily without withdrawal symptoms, but only if they *want* to stop. Perhaps you have heard the old joke: How many psychiatrists does it take to change a light bulb? The answer is? Only one, but only if the light bulb *wants* to change.

Hypnosis is *not* about the hypnotist exercising his or her control or "mental powers" over the person who is the hypnotic subject. Hypnosis, in truth, is about learning to exercise more control over yourself, your experience, and your behavior. Hypnosis is really about being helped to tap your own untapped inner strengths and resources so that you can have increased *self-control.*

**Hypnotized Individuals Cannot Be Made to Bark Like a Dog.** "So," you may ask, "how do you explain why people do such silly things in hypnosis stage shows?" If you have seen such a show, you may have seen people acting as if they were a dog, a chicken, a person of the opposite sex, and so on, when the hypnotist gives them the command.

Believe me, human nature being what it is, people always do things for a reason. The context of the show (acting zany or silly or absurdly, acting hypnotized and having fun) gives the volunteer participants a sort of "license" to act out in outlandish ways, and let themselves go. It is considered acceptable to go along with the hypnotist's outrageous commands for entertainment purposes.

Most onlookers also are unaware that stage hypnotists screen their volunteers for their heightened suggestibility and willingness to comply with the hypnotist's commands and suggestions. Stage hypnotists also frequently have previously trained accomplices or "shills" in the audience, and they are good at selecting only those new participants who will be cooperative. Members of the audience who want to be part of the show and who have possible exhibitionist tendencies make the best subjects for entertainment purposes.

**You Cannot Lose Control or Go Crazy in Hypnosis.** You cannot lose control or go crazy in hypnosis, provided that you are not on the verge of having a breakdown or losing control of yourself in the first place. Anyone who is mentally or psychiatrically unstable should not use hypnosis unless they are under the care of a qualified mental-health professional who is employing hypnosis as a treatment tool in their care. If you were in such a mentally unstable state, the rule of thumb is that you should get yourself to a hospital emergency room, psychiatric hospital, or police station as soon as possible. If such were the case, you would want to be safely contained where you would be safe from yourself, safe from others, and others would be safe from you!

Hypnosis is not like alcohol or certain drugs that lessens some people's inhibitions to the point where they might be more likely to do something crazy. Even in those situations, persons sometimes consciously or unconsciously use alcohol or drugs as an excuse to let their "wilder side" have a night out. That is just not what hypnosis is about. Sometimes people in hypnosis recall forgotten or repressed memories, but the fact that such memories are recalled does not imply that they are accurate or factual. You need independent corroboration to establish their accuracy or truth.

**Hypnosis Is Not a Truth Serum.** Finally, hypnosis is not a truth serum. Also, when you are in hypnosis, you cannot be compelled to say or blurt out things that you do not want to share. You retain control at all times.

# ◎ Hypnosis Is a State and a Procedure

In defining what "hypnosis" is, we first need to distinguish between the hypnotic state of consciousness, and the method or procedure that is employed for inducing or producing this particular altered state. These are often confused by interchangeably calling both of them simply "hypnosis." Because the use of the blanket term "hypnosis" can be confusing, I will clarify the way I use the terms now, before we go on.

The method or procedure for inducing or producing the hypnotic state is technically called a *hypnotic induction method*. The mental state induced through the employment of a hypnotic induction method is called the *hypnotic trance state*. There are hundreds of different hypnotic induction methods. Many books have been written that are devoted entirely to the induction of hypnosis. In chapter 4, I describe eight simple and useful hypnotic induction methods for helping yourself into hypnosis. One or more of them is right for you.

When you seek treatment from a health professional who uses hypnosis clinically, then that professional's use of hypnosis is termed *clinical hypnosis*. When someone else helps you enter, or induce, the hypnotic state, it is technically called *hetero-hypnosis*. When you do it yourself, it is called *self-hypnosis*. Irrespective of whether someone else helps you to enter the hypnotic state, or you do it yourself, the method used to enter hypnosis is called an *induction*, or *hypnotic induction*. If you employ an induction to help yourself into hypnosis, this is called *self-hypnosis* or a *self-hypnosis induction*.

# ◎ My Definition of Hypnosis

But we haven't yet actually defined "hypnosis" have we? Here is my simple and concise definition of hypnosis. It emphasizes the key ingredients that make hypnosis such an effective treatment for relieving pain.

*"Hypnosis" or "hypnotic trance" is an altered state of consciousness that involves comfortable relaxation, a redirection of attention, and active sensory imagination. It is a special state of resting alertness. While a person is in this altered state, that person's focus of attention can be redirected to what is important for the purpose at hand.*

The term "altered state of consciousness" bears explanation. The hypnosis altered state is unique but natural. It is induced whenever the unconscious or subconscious mind is alerted to pay attention to a unique form of communication. This spontaneously produces a divided state of attention or consciousness.

So you may wonder, how is your attention divided? The answer is that your conscious mind is pleasantly absorbed in relaxing, enjoyable sensations, a pleasant memory, or an imaginative fantasy while your unconscious attends to the communication that initiated or continues to maintain the hypnosis altered state.

It is like you are *here* and *there* at the same time. Your conscious mind may be on the beach (or wherever your favorite place is), but your unconscious is functioning like a "hidden observer" (Hilgard and Hilgard 1996). Now here's the clincher: to the degree that the initiating communication (the hypnosis induction) is compelling, engaging, and absorbing, the division or split in consciousness is heightened or deepened. And the deeper the split in consciousness is, the more your unconscious or hidden observer is awakened and responsive to the initiating hypnotic communication!

When your unconscious is very responsive, your responses to hypnotic suggestions feel automatic, spontaneous, and involuntary. They just happen easily and comfortably with little or no conscious deliberation. So when you begin to learn and experience self-hypnosis in chapter 4, you will have a range of responses. The depth of the division in your consciousness will vary. But what is most important is not the *depth* of this division or split, but rather the *quality* of your experience.

You will be able to choose the self-hypnosis induction that is best for you. Because it is your choice, it will be a good quality experience.

**A Focusing Mechanism.** Hypnosis is also a focusing mechanism and a way of communicating precisely with your *unconscious, subconscious,* or *inner mind.* All three of these terms are different names for the same thing. They are generally employed interchangeably, and I will follow this convention throughout the rest of this book.

When your body is comfortably relaxed and at ease and your conscious mind is absorbed in an interesting experience involving compelling sensory imagery, your inner mind or unconscious mind is alerted to pay attention. This frees your inner mind to be open and receptive to acceptable positive ideas and suggestions. Once your inner mind accepts an idea, it transforms that idea into a reality. This can help you change your experience in the way that you desire.

**All Hypnosis Is Really Self-Hypnosis.** You may find it surprising that all hypnosis is really self-hypnosis. That is because, while you can be given positive suggestions for change, in order for that change to occur, you must accept those suggestions and make them your own. So, all suggestions that you accept become self-suggestions.

Hypnosis and self-hypnosis are simply tools for making positive changes more easily and quickly. However, like any other tool, these tools can be used correctly or incorrectly. When they are used correctly, their positive benefits become quite evident. When we learn how to use self-hypnosis correctly, we begin to notice positive changes in our thinking, feeling, behaving, and experience. When we use it incorrectly, we simply fail to produce the results we intend or desire. In part 2, I will teach you how to use this tool effectively.

Hypnosis is easier than you may think. The induction of self-hypnosis first involves resting, giving yourself permission to be at ease, and letting go of tensions. While you restfully ease into relaxation *without* falling asleep, you become absorbed in your pleasant experience and redirect your focus of attention.

As you easily and comfortably become absorbed in what you are paying attention to, you begin to experience a suspension of your habitual critical judgment. In other words, your "inner critic" temporarily shuts down or quiets. This leads to a feeling of relative effortlessness as your responses become relatively automatic.

While you are in this altered state, the doorway to the unconscious opens, and with your conscious permission, your unconscious becomes receptive to the information it needs to change the experience or behavior you want to change. Once the unconscious accepts this information, it can't ignore it. It must act on it and begin to change what it is about yourself that you want to change (Zarren and Eimer 2001).

**A Three-Step Process.** The first step in learning self-hypnosis is to be guided into hypnosis by someone who understands how to communicate with the unconscious mind and who also is experienced in practicing self-hypnosis. This would be an experienced and well-trained health-care professional who has also been trained in the clinical and personal use of hypnosis. In this case, that is me! The second step is to be taught how to repeat the process on your own. The third step is to practice, practice, practice so as to imprint the experience in your unconscious. We will do this in chapter 4.

**EASING into the Hypnotic State.** Once you know how, self-hypnosis involves:

1.  **E**asily resting and relaxing;

2.  **A**bsorbing yourself in a neutral or pleasant experience by focusing your attention;

3.  **S**uspending your critical thinking temporarily;

4.  **I**nterrupting your usual conscious orientation to time, space, your body, and yourself;

5.  **N**ot trying to make anything happen, or exerting any notable conscious effort;

6.  **G**etting more and more comfortable and enjoying the experience.

See how easy it is!

# ◎ Hypnotic Analgesia

When either hypnosis or self-hypnosis is utilized to produce pain relief, it's known as *hypnotic analgesia*. Hypnotic analgesia employs hypnotic suggestions to reduce the felt intensity of pain. I am talking about EASING into an altered, neutral state or an altered state of pleasure. Remember that pleasure is the opposite of pain. A "persistent pain state" is characterized by opposing qualities to those involved in EASING into self-hypnosis.

For example, in a persistent pain state, a person feels:

1.  *Strained, tense, and uncomfortable* as opposed to **E**asy, *relaxed, and comfortable*;

2.  *Scattered and distractible* as opposed to **A**bsorbed and focused;

3. *Critical and vigilant* as opposed to **S**uspending criticism and judgments;

4. *Trapped* as opposed to feeling **I**n control and in charge;

5. *That he or she has to try hard to not be in pain, or escape,* as opposed to **N**ot trying.

6. *More and more uncomfortable* versus feeling that he or she is **G**etting more comfortable.

This is why, when it comes to relieving pain, hypnosis is a great tool! You will learn how to use it to hypnotize yourself out of pain in part 2.

# ◎ Hypnotic Suggestion

When we talk about hypnotic suggestion, we have to distinguish between suggestions as ideas and the process of giving yourself or others suggestions. A *positive suggestion* is an idea that automatically creates the expectation that you are going to feel a positive change in your experience. You expect it to happen. You feel it and know it, and there is no doubt.

The process of suggestion is the means of making this happen. It involves establishing an image in your unconscious mind of a specific idea, action, feeling, or experience so that the desired change can take place. You don't have to be in a hypnotic trance state to benefit from positive suggestion. For example, can you recall a time when your doctor prescribed a remedy and told you something like, "This is a very effective (or powerful) medicine," or, "This medicine will really work." Did you experience some relief? Your doctor was capitalizing on the power of positive suggestion.

The value of hypnosis is that when you're in a hypnotic trance state, your expectation of positive changes in feelings and experience and behavior automatically leads to the realization of those changes. Once you learn how to enter and exit self-hypnosis, you will be able to use this skill to change your experience of pain. You will expect to feel more comfortable. Then, when you enter self-hypnosis, your mental expectation of increased comfort will be transformed into increased comfort in reality.

## A Definition of Suggestion

A *suggestion* is the transmission of an idea by one person (or it could be a company advertisement, or even a book, such as this book!) to another person with the intention of automatically, spontaneously, and unconsciously affecting the recipient's actions, motivations, and experience. This happens without any or much conscious deliberation by the recipient. The recipient is open to the suggestion to the degree to which they are receptive toward the expressed wishes or direct or implied directives of the sender.

Suggestion depends upon adequate rapport and is different from arbitrary commands. *Rapport* means being in harmony with the person delivering the suggestions. It means feeling an affinity for that person. It requires that you feel understood. Hopefully, by this point, we have rapport, and you feel that I understand what it is like to have chronic pain.

# ◎ Hypnosis and Memory

Human brain cells, or neurons, retain and recall specific images long after a person has actually seen, heard, felt, smelled, or tasted the actual object of experience. The amazing brain appears to have a system of calling up and replaying the same cellular event that fired up at the time of the original experience and that led to the initial formation of the memory. Apparently, this system is reinforced and strengthened by repetition and practice. Therefore, by using our memories, we can keep them from getting "rusty." I say, memories, plural, because we have different memory systems for different sensations and experiences. Hypnosis involves recalling pleasant experiences, memories, and images and becoming absorbed in them.

When you get into the habit of making pain-relieving, pleasurable, and comforting images in your mind's eye, you actually fool your brain into believing that those images are real. Then your brain begins to get into the habit of creating those feelings and strengthening those memories. On the other hand, maintaining the habit of thinking repeatedly about pain and discomfort keeps the brain stuck in the habit of generating negative images and memories. Remember the pain neuro-matrix, that vicious pain cycle in the nervous system that we discussed in chapter 1? Our goal is to close the pain gate and imprint a "comfort neuro-matrix" or "comfort cycle."

# ◎ Sensory Memory Systems and Active Sensory Imagination

People differ in terms of which memory systems are strongest for them. Different sensations can be recalled in differing degrees of intensity and vividness; sights, sounds, smells, tastes, touch, pressure, movement, and so on. For some people, visually recalling pleasant sights is what's most compelling and absorbing. Other people respond more strongly to the memory of sounds, such as being at a great concert or having a good conversation. Still other people become most engaged when they remember scents and/ or flavors, such as when I recall the scent and flavor of my grandmother's freshly baked bread and cookies right out of the oven.

Take a moment to consider what positive sensory impressions are most pleasant and compelling for you. What comes to mind?

Other physical feelings that some people can become actively absorbed in recalling are movement and touch. For example, you can become actively involved in recalling the physical feelings associated with the last time you took a good walk, went swimming, went skiing, played tennis, laid on the warm sand on the beach, experienced the sensual touch of a lover, or had a great meal. Many people find that they can become most absorbed in a memory by recalling multiple sensory impressions; feelings, scents, sights, sounds, flavors and so on.

Active sensory imagination refers to the deliberate and conscious, or spontaneous and unconscious, recall of sensory impressions and experiences. This is an important part of self-hypnosis. So, how does this apply to controlling your pain? It applies because, on one level, *pain* is just a *sensation*. While in actuality, pain is a lot more than just a sensation (it's an unpleasant experience), the fact that we can look at pain as just a sensation is a real advantage. It makes pain amenable to being changed. That is because no sensations are permanent, and all sensations can be changed. Active sensory imagination is one means of changing sensations.

The fact that pain is also a lot more than just a sensation is also an advantage. It makes pain amenable to methods of alleviation other than those that are just physical methods.

Research has shown that, under the right conditions, hypnosis is one of the most effective psychological, nondrug methods of relieving and controlling pain. The "right conditions" means adequate mental and psychological preparation. By reading as far as you have and continuing to read on, you are being mentally and psychologically prepared to develop the necessary skills for hypnotizing yourself out of unnecessary and dysfunctional pain.

**Alert Hypnosis.** As mentioned earlier, self-relaxation is an important part of entering and enjoying the hypnotic state. When you're relaxed, you cannot be uncomfortable! Relaxation is good for us and an antidote to pain. Additionally, most people can become focused and enter what is called "alert hypnosis" by becoming actively mentally and/or physically involved in an activity without relaxation. For example, can you remember the last time you were totally, pleasantly, and actively absorbed in a physical or mental activity? Depending on your interests, talents, and schedule, that might have been while playing a sport, exercising, studying, doing your job, or working at a hobby. You probably were calm but alert and focused and "in the flow." Were you feeling alert or deeply relaxed? Can you remember if you felt in a lot of pain at the time?

I would guess that your absorption in what you were doing limited the extent to which you were paying attention to your pain, as everpresent as it might be. Even if you recall that you had just a few minutes of relative comfort, isn't that better than no comfort at all?

Perhaps your pain limited how long you could stay absorbed in your activity. I wouldn't be surprised if this was the case. Pain has a way of breaking through. I have to take frequent breaks from writing to stretch, relax, and breathe or else I experience greater breakthrough pain than I typically do anyway. I try to take my breaks before the pain breaks through and forces me to stop what I'm doing. However, being human, sometimes I forget. Then I pay for it.

What all of this leads to is some exercises designed to help you explore your active sensory imagination so that you can discover which sensory memory systems are most compelling and absorbing for you. These are the systems that you will find most helpful for inducing and utilizing self-hypnosis to change your pain experience.

# Exercise 3.1: Exploring Your Active Sensory Imagination

I am going to use the term *visualization* to refer to your use of any kind of sensory imagery that you experience as compelling, absorbing, and engaging. This is one of the activities that leads to increased suggestibility and the altered state of consciousness we call hypnosis. It's also one of the building blocks of hypnotic analgesia. So let's explore your sensory imagination abilities. Find a quiet, comfortable place where you can focus and remain undisturbed for around fifteen minutes so that you can do the following exercise.

## Instructions

There are a number of "Is it possible?" questions below. Each question, along with the included suggestions, is designed to help you check out your ability to remember experiences that emphasize a particular sensory system. As you read each question, permit yourself to have an open, receptive, and curious frame of mind. Exercise your active imagination and allow yourself to become absorbed in your experience.

After you read each "Is it possible?" question below and the associated suggestions, you can respond to them with your eyes open, or if you prefer, you can sit back with your eyes closed and experience your responses.

**Sounds.** Is it possible for you to hear the sounds in your mind of some marvelous something that happened to you in the past? Consider something that gave you great pleasure. It might have been a concert, or a play, or a movie, a tape or CD, or a conversation you had. Is it possible for you to bring back that experience in your head and actually hear it all over again now, almost as if you are there and it is happening now? Take all the time you need to do this. Permit yourself to become absorbed and enjoy any other pleasurable sensations you happen to notice as you do this exercise. If you found this easy, you are especially responsive to auditory (sound) sensory impressions and experiences. Choosing a self-hypnosis induction method that utilizes this sense will be particularly helpful for you.

**Scents.** Is it possible for you to remember a scent or aroma that gives you great pleasure? Can you bring back in full detail in your head and in your nose an experience that happened to you recently or some time ago that involved that pleasant and satisfying scent? Is it possible for you to actually smell that scent all over again, almost as if you are there and its aroma is around you now? Take all the time you need. Permit yourself to become absorbed and enjoy any other pleasurable sensations you happen to notice as you do this exercise. If you found this easy, you are especially responsive to sensory impressions of aromatic scents. It will be particularly helpful for you to incorporate this sense into your self-hypnosis experience, as it will make this experience more vivid and absorbing.

**Feelings.** Is it possible for you to remember a pleasant experience that happened to you some time ago and really feel that experience in terms of how your body felt? And also, are there specific emotions involved, like satisfaction or pleasure? Is it possible for you to bring back those emotional and bodily feelings and sensations and experience them all over again now, almost as if you are there, and it's happening, and you're experiencing it now? Take all the time you need to do this. Permit yourself to become absorbed in and enjoy any other pleasurable sensations you happen to notice as you do this exercise. If you found this easy, you are especially responsive to tactile, kinesthetic, and emotional sensory impressions and experiences. Choosing a hypnotic induction method that utilizes this sense will be particularly helpful for you. Remember that pain is a kinesthetic and tactile sensation among other things.

**Sights.** Is it possible for you to bring back visually the memory of a place you visited some time in the past that you really enjoyed? Is it possible for you to begin to see the sights associated with that experience and the specific images and details? The colors? The shapes? The textures and the shades associated with that place? Is it possible for you to do that comfortably in your head and actually see that place all over again, almost as if you're there now? Take as much time as you need to do this. Permit yourself to become absorbed in and enjoy any other pleasurable sensations you happen to notice as you do this exercise. If you found this easy, you are especially responsive to visual sensory impressions and images. Choosing a hypnotic induction method that utilizes this sense will be particularly helpful for you.

**Flavors and Tastes.** Is it possible for you to remember a particularly pleasant or delicious flavor or taste? Can you bring back in full detail in your head and in your mouth an experience that happened to you, recently or some time ago, that involved that pleasant, delicious, and satisfying flavor or taste? Is it possible for you to remember the taste or flavor that experience left in your mouth and actually taste that good flavor all over again now, almost as if you're there, and it is happening now? Take all the time you need to do this. Permit yourself to become absorbed in and enjoy any other pleasurable sensations you happen to notice. If you found this easy, you are especially responsive to memories and impressions of tastes and flavors. It might be helpful for you to incorporate this sense into your self-hypnosis experience.

**Multisensory Recall.** Is it possible for you to imagine a pleasant place that's very special to you? A place you've been to before and would like to go to again? Or perhaps a place you've always wanted to visit? Can you experience your place as if you're there now? Can you become more relaxed and comfortable and go deeper into your experience? Do you begin to see clearly the images associated with that place— the colors, the shapes, the textures, and the shades associated with it? Is it possible for you to begin to feel the way that place made you feel? The experience of being there and the satisfaction and pleasure of that particular experience in terms of how your body felt? And in terms of the emotions and feelings attached to that experience? Can you hear the sounds associated with that place, bringing back that experience in your head and actually hearing it all over again? And can you remember the particular scents associated with that place, bring back that experience in your head, and smell them all over again? Can you remember the flavors that the experience left in your mouth and taste it, too?

The more sensory impressions, images, and experiences you were able to recall, the more flexibility this gives you in using your imagination to reduce pain. You'll have more choices. For example, if you feel uncomfortable before falling asleep, you may simply have to decide if you are going to imagine yourself floating in a calm ocean or floating in space. You may wish to choose between imagining yourself lying on a warm beach or cozying up to a warm fireplace in the middle of winter. The point is to use all of your compelling and engaging senses to create a pleasant and absorbing experience.

It can be helpful to ask yourself which types of sensory impressions were most vivid, intense, and pleasant and which felt most real for you. Usually we have one or two sensory systems that are more powerful and evocative than others. These sensory representational systems, or *visualization abilities*, are our primary or preferred ways of perceiving and recalling experiences. Therefore, they can be called our *lead*, *primary*, or *preferred* sensory systems. It is helpful to know what they are because this will inform you about the easiest ways to actively employ your sensory imagination to enter the altered state of consciousness we call hypnosis.

If you found several types of sensory imagery compelling and absorbing (multisensory recall), as I stated earlier, this fact will enhance your flexibility and openness to benefitting from various hypnotic and nonhypnotic coping methods. You can choose the hypnotic coping strategies that are most relevant, feel the most natural, and that appeal to you the most.

# ◎ Reading into Self-Hypnosis

Most of us have had the experience at one time or another of reading ourselves to sleep. You know the feeling. You are sitting in a comfortable chair, or lying in bed reading. As you continue to read, your eyes start to feel tired, your eyelids start to feel heavier and blink more frequently. You start to read word by word, and the same things over again. Soon it becomes a struggle to keep your eyes open! Your eyes begin to close all by themselves, and you fall into a restful, comfortable, very well-earned and deserved sleep state.

The following exercise will give you the experience of reading yourself into self-hypnosis and relaxation. However, as I explained earlier, hypnosis and self-hypnosis are not the same altered state of consciousness as sleep. The only basic similarity is that both altered states are entered into easily and effortlessly. You can try to fall asleep, but that is NOT the way you fall asleep. It is counterproductive to try, or work hard, to fall asleep. Similarly, you need not try, or work hard, to enter self-hypnosis. Just think and imagine along with the instructions and suggestions that I give you as you read them, and your self-hypnosis experiences will be easy, effortless, pleasant, and worthwhile.

## Exercise 3.2: Read Yourself into Self-Hypnosis

Silently read the indented paragraph below very slowly in your head. Read one word every three seconds. Stop after you read each word. Then start reading again, continuing with the next word. Keep your head as still as you can. Just move your eyes. You may not get to read all of the paragraph because soon after you start reading that paragraph slowly like this, your eyes will grow tired, and you will want to close them. You will then enter a comfortable state of self-relaxation and self-hypnosis after you close your eyes. Stay in relaxation and hypnosis, remaining quiet for a short while. When you're ready to awaken, count up to five and then open your eyes. At five, you will be awake, and yet remain comfortable and relaxed at the same time.

Now start reading slowly, word by word:

> *You can close your eyes and enter hypnosis after you have read twenty-three to thirty-seven words. When your eyes feel tired, close them. When you close your eyes, you will enter relaxation and hypnosis, and remain quiet. Your unconscious mind is receptive to all of the words you read in this paragraph. You remember how pleasant it feels to be very comfortably relaxed and quiet. When you're ready to end your hypnosis, you can return to an awake and alert state by counting from one to five. At five, you will be awake, and yet comfortable and relaxed at the same time. If you have read this far, close your eyes and enter relaxation and hypnosis now.*

What were the results of your checking out your ability to read yourself into self-relaxation and hypnosis? What was the experience like for you?

1.  Did you close your eyes and enter relaxation and hypnosis before you finished reading the above paragraph? If you did, then you will probably be able to enter self-hypnosis very easily while you read the instructions for doing the self-hypnosis exercises in the following chapters.

2.  Did you close your eyes and enter relaxation and hypnosis after you finished reading the entire paragraph? If this is what you experienced, you may find it easier to do the following self-hypnosis exercises after you've read through each exercise one or more times first. Then, you will be able to enter self-hypnosis easily while you read the instructions.

3.  If you did not feel that you entered self-hypnosis and relaxation yet, you will in the exercises to follow. The exercise you just did primed and prepared you to ease into self-hypnosis when you do one or more of the exercises in the next chapter. You may wish to record some additional notes now in your notebook about your experience for later reference.

Remember: This book is written for everyone who is in pain and wants relief! The only requirement on your part is an unequivocally positive answer to the question I asked you earlier, which was, "Do I want to feel better?"

# Part Two

## How to Hypnotize Yourself Out of Pain Now

*The heart of the wise teaches his mouth, and adds learning to his lips.*

**—Proverbs 16:23**

*But blessed are your eyes for they see, and your ears for they hear; for assuredly, I say to you that many prophets and righteous men desired to see what you see, and did not see it, and hear what you hear, and did not hear it.*

**—Matthew 13:16–17**

# FOUR

## Practice Inducing Self-Hypnosis

*Suggestions involving a need to remember sensory stimuli and sequences of events are part of most hypnotic induction rituals . . . An hypnoidal state is entered when recalling a tune, remembering the visual images of waves breaking on the beach, the movements of a candle flame, and the words of a poem . . .*

**—David B. Cheek, M.D.**

The first thing I would like you to do is just experience the pleasure of repeatedly entering and exiting the self-hypnosis trance state. In order to do that, you will need to choose a self-hypnosis induction method that appeals to you—it's your choice.

With this goal in mind, I describe eight self-hypnosis induction methods below. I invite you to explore all of them and then choose to practice the *one* you like the best. Once you choose that one method, stick with it. Spend a week or so practicing the method twice a day for about ten to fifteen minutes each time. Ideally, this should be once in the morning, some time before eating breakfast, and once in the late afternoon or early evening, before eating supper. However, there is no need to be rigid about these times. It's simply best to do self-hypnosis when you are neither full nor very hungry, so that you can concentrate.

# ◎ Your First Goal

My first goal for you is simply to imprint the experience in your unconscious of entering and exiting self-hypnosis and self-relaxation—nothing more and nothing less. But please heed this:

**Warning:** You should only practice self-hypnosis when and where it is safe and appropriate for you to do so. This would be in a place where you will be undisturbed for fifteen to twenty minutes. **You should never practice self-hypnosis, self-relaxation, or any other inner-focusing methods while you are operating dangerous machinery such as a motor vehicle.** You should simply never practice self-hypnosis when you need to be alert and responsive to external events, other people, etc. Doing otherwise is likely to be extremely dangerous to both yourself and others.

**A Pertinent Reminder.** Persistent pain is primarily *kinesthetic* (physical) and *internal* (within you and your body). Therefore, one of the things we want to eventually accomplish is to *externalize* your pain sensations, that is, get them out of you. Another thing we want to accomplish is to substitute more pleasant kinesthetic physical sensations for the unpleasant ones.

The information in chapter 3 enabled you to explore your active sensory imagination skills and learn about your primary sensory memory systems. Hopefully, working through that chapter gave you insight about the sensory memory systems that are most compelling and absorbing for you.

If you found that one of your dominant sensory systems is tactile-kinesthetic (your sense of touch and physical, bodily feelings), then a tactile-kinesthetic method of inducing self-hypnosis may appeal to you. If you are predominantly visual, then a procedure that primarily relies on visual attention and eye fixation may work best. Explore all the following methods and choose the one that works best for you.

# ◎ Sitting Yourself Down Comfortably

For this exercise and all of the self-hypnosis exercises to follow that involve reading yourself into self-hypnosis, you will need to situate yourself so that you are comfortable and so that you can turn the pages of this book without disturbing your level of relaxation or trance. In fact, when you are situated comfortably and are absorbed in your self-hypnosis experience, you will become more absorbed and go deeper into self-hypnosis each time you turn a page.

So, sit comfortably with your back, head, and neck supported and your feet resting either flat on the floor or on a foot rest. It will be very helpful if you can prop this book up in front of you in some way so that you can read easily and turn the pages effortlessly. You want to have your book propped up high enough so that you do not have to look down too much.

One way to accomplish this is to sit upright at a table or desk with this book propped up in front of you on a stand of some type and your hands resting palms facing down on the table on either side of this book. To do this, you can pile some other books up and lean this book against them, or you can obtain or devise a book stand.

Another way to have the book accessible is to sit in a comfortable chair with your hands resting palms down on your thighs, or possibly on the arm rests of the chair, if the chair has arm rests and this is comfortable. Either way is fine. You will want to have your book propped up in front of you, either on a separate stand, a height-adjustable table, a lap desk, or on a pillow or several pillows. If you use a lap desk or a pillow, it may be most comfortable to rest your hands palms down on the lap desk or pillow on either side of your book, depending of course on the size of your lap desk or pillow.

## Self-Hypnosis Method 1:
## Zarren's Marble Method

The first induction method we are going to explore is "Zarren's Marble Method" (Zarren and Eimer 2001). It is an ideal method for externalizing physical discomfort and negative thoughts and feelings. It combines *visual* and *tactile-kinesthetic* sensory systems, and redirects your focus of attention away from your pain and other physical symptoms. This method provides a source of neutral, pleasant, visual and tactile-kinesthetic counter-stimulation that can temporarily inhibit or lessen the negative stimulation of pain. This counterstimulation comes from holding, manipulating, and concentrating on a marble.

You will need to obtain a medium-sized marble such as can be purchased at most toy or game stores or at a magic shop. A marble is an ideal object because it is smooth, round, shiny, and interesting. However, if you are unable to get your hands on a marble, you may substitute another small, firm, interesting object that you can manipulate in one hand.

For example, one of those oval or circular, flat, clear or colored, smooth, decorative glass marbles that are often used to fill vases will work. You also may choose to use a small mineral rock (such as a piece of rose quartz or amethyst) or a smooth pebble that is at least three-quarters of an inch wide and long, so that you can manipulate it easily and comfortably with one hand. A metal or wooden key ring, a chain or amulet, or piece of jewelry can also work.

The point is that, if you can't get a marble, you want to choose an object that you can look at, hold in your hand, manipulate, and that you find pleasing and interesting. It should be something that you will enjoy looking at and holding and that you can concentrate on, something that you can feel good about making special and your own.

## Instructions for Using the Script Below.

I've worded the script below based on the assumption that you are using a marble, which is the best choice of object to hold onto. Read each numbered set of instructions while you hold your marble in you hand. After you have read each set of instructions, do what is asked, and let yourself experience what is suggested. Then read the next set of instructions. Continue in this manner until you come to the end of the procedure. Each time you turn a page, you will become more absorbed and go deeper into self-relaxation and self-hypnosis. This exercise should take about ten to fifteen minutes. You can repeat the entire procedure several times in this way until you know it. Then you will be able to do the entire thing in one smooth flow without having to read or think about each step.

> Begin by choosing a marble that feels comfortable, that you would like to keep as your own. Marbles come in many different sizes, colors, and textures. All of them can be very beautiful. So, sit back in a chair with the marble you have chosen in your hand and notice that just holding your marble brings a smile to your lips and a nice feeling inside of you. Marbles instantly take us back to a childhood time when we were enjoying ourselves.

Follow the above instructions now, and then read on.

> Hold your marble between your thumb and fingers and feel it by rolling it around. Look at your marble and notice its colors and pattern. Notice the way the light changes the colors embedded in the marble. Keep looking at your marble as you roll it around in your hand. Feel the slight imperfections in the round glass globe. Realize that something this beautiful doesn't have to be perfect and yet still can be very special.

Follow the above instructions now, then read the next set of instructions, which leads to closing your eyes. This next set of instructions also tells you what to do after you close your eyes.

*As you continue to look at your marble and roll it around in your hand, notice how much more relaxed you feel. Notice how, as you continue to stare at the marble, your eyelids are blinking more frequently than usual. When your eyelids get very heavy, or when the marble begins to go out of focus, gently close your eyes and close your hand around the marble so that it doesn't fall out of your hand. You will immediately go deeply into relaxation. After you close your eyes, pay attention to the feel of the marble in your hand. Notice how much warmer the marble feels and if you can, see in your mind's eye the changing swirls of color in your marble. Continue to concentrate on the marble and permit yourself to go deeper into relaxation and hypnosis. If your mind wanders, the moment you realize you're thinking of something different, just bring your mind back to concentrating on the marble in your hand. After a little while, blink your eyes and open them wide.*

Now follow the above instructions that you've just read and then read on.

*You control your marble. You're in charge of it, and the marble helps you to experience deep relaxation without pressure or tension or stress. It helps you to feel very comfortable. Just holding the marble can help you to feel very comfortable. The next time you close your eyes, your concentration on the marble will be even stronger and your feeling of relaxation will be even deeper. When you are relaxed, you cannot be angry or anxious, and you cannot be uncomfortable. These are emotional and physical opposites of each other. Relaxation is your first goal, leading to changes in how you feel, think, and behave. You're building a memory of deep relaxation you can use to help yourself relax on your own.*

Close your eyes again and resume concentrating on the marble for a minute or two. Then blink your eyes, open them wide, and read on.

*Plan to use your marble a few times a day to relax yourself. Hold the marble in your hand, look at it, roll it between your thumb and fingers, feel it, see the colors change, the reflecting light, and relax. Close your eyes gently, close your hand around the marble, and relax much deeper. Stay in relaxation for a while and enjoy your freedom from physical and emotional discomfort. Then, when your deepest mind is fully aware of how much comfort you have and knows it can maintain that comfort for some time after you awaken yourself from self-hypnosis, turn your hand face up, and slowly open your hand. Blink your eyes, open them wide, and come back fully alert, sound in mind, sound in body, and in control of your feelings.*

Now continue to concentrate on the feel of the marble in your hand and read on.

*In addition to using the marble to help yourself go deeply into relaxation, from now on you will be able to use this marble to relax yourself, in seconds, whenever you need to most, wherever you are, without closing your eyes, and without anyone knowing you are doing it. Just holding the marble in your hand will bring back a feeling of relaxation. This almost instant relaxation method is a very valuable tool that you can have available to deal with stressful situations no matter when or where they may occur. Now close your eyes again and continue to concentrate on the marble for a few more minutes. Then, when your deepest mind is fully aware of how much comfort you have now and knows it can maintain that comfort and continue to process what we have accomplished in this exercise, turn your hand face up and slowly open your hand. Blink your eyes, open them wide, and come back fully alert, sound in mind, sound in body, and in control of your feelings.*

## Self-Hypnosis Method 2:
## Eye Fixation, Attention-to-Breathing Method

The following self-hypnosis induction method is brief, direct, and conducive to producing a physiologically calm and relaxed state. It redirects your attention internally to your breathing. So it is a kinesthetic induction. But it is a visual method also, because it also has you focusing your visual attention while you are paying attention to your breathing.

**Your Breathing Is Your Road to Relaxation.** Your breathing is a physical reflection of your relative state of calm versus arousal. When you are calm, relaxed, and feeling restful, your breathing tends to be slow and regular, even and rhythmic. When you are in this state, you naturally tend to breathe more from your diaphragm and belly and less from your upper chest, upper back, and shoulders. Breathing from your diaphragm is easier on your back and neck and also a more natural and comfortable way to breathe.

On the other hand, when you are not calm, but restless, clammed up, nervous, anxious, tense, or in a lot of pain, your breathing tends to reflect this also. Your breathing tends to be uneven, labored, shallow, quicker, and more irregular. It also tends to come more from your chest, upper back, and shoulders. You even may gasp for and swallow air.

When you're feeling relaxed and breathing calmly, you cannot at the same time be clammed up, tense, stressed, and breathing nervously, because they are opposite physiological states. Your breathing reflects the status of your nervous system: calm versus aroused, relaxed versus tense. By slowing down your breathing and breathing calmly, evenly, and easily, you can induce a state of relaxation and calm.

When you concentrate on your breathing without trying to change your breathing, the normal rhythm of your breathing begins to exert a natural calming effect on your mind and body. As you become increasingly absorbed in the natural rhythm of your calm, easy breathing, you ease into self-hypnosis trance. Your breathing really is the "royal road to relaxation and calm."

The following self-hypnosis method will enable you to *read yourself into self-hypnosis and relaxation*. This exercise focuses on helping you attain a calm and restful physiological state primarily through concentration on your breathing without consciously trying to change your breathing.

### *Instructions for Using the Script Below.*

The script below is best employed as follows:

First read through the entire script once or twice to get the gist of the method. Then begin reading the script a third time. You are going to read yourself into self-hypnosis. Keep your head  still, and just move your eyes as you read s-l-o-w-l-y, either silently or quietly aloud in a relaxed voice. Eventually, your eyes will grow tired and heavy. In this exercise, you should read on, even as you get sleepy. You may find from time to time that you are reading some of the same words over again. That is all right. Just keep reading to the end of the induction. By using the script in this way, you will experience the intended effects of the exercise and learn this calming self-hypnosis induction method.

Each time you turn a page, you will become more absorbed and go deeper into self-relaxation and self-hypnosis. You will also go deeper into self-relaxation with each word you read, and if you read aloud, with the sound of your own voice.

Read these words slowly, a few words at a time. Sit comfortably in a chair, your feet flat on the floor, your arms and hands resting comfortably with the palms down, and your head still. As you move your eyes slowly from one group of words to the next, also pay attention to your breathing without trying to change your breathing. Just let yourself breathe normally while you pay attention to your breathing and continue reading slowly.

*Let your breathing become the center of your thoughts and attention while your eyes stay focused on slowly reading the words on the page in front of you. If your mind wanders, and it may, the moment you realize that you are thinking of something else, bring your mind back to your reading and to concentrating on your breathing.*

*As you do this, you will notice that your eyelids begin to blink more frequently than usual, and they may feel heavier. This more frequent blinking and the way your eyelids feel are a part of this self-hypnosis experience and are a result of how and what you're reading. Shortly, you will find that your eyes want to close. However, keep your eyes open and continue reading. Later, when you do this exercise on your own without reading, you can close your eyes comfortably. But for right now, you will do best by keeping your eyes open so that you can keep reading. Also, any fluttering of your eyelids is a normal part of the self-hypnosis experience. After a while, you will pay no attention to any fluttering you may experience.*

*Meanwhile, your breathing begins to change as you become more relaxed. Notice how comfortable your breathing feels and how much more relaxed you have become. Make sure to keep reading S-L-O-W-L-Y. Allow your more comfortable breathing to take you deeper into relaxation and hypnosis, deeper with each breath that you take, and deeper with each word that you read regardless of the meaning of the words. As you go deeper and deeper into relaxation and hypnosis with each breath and each word, the doorway to your unconscious opens. With your permission, I have the opportunity to talk to your unconscious and give it information it needs to help you learn to use self-hypnosis well to feel more comfortable.*

*By doing this exercise, you are learning what it feels like to be comfortably relaxed. You are building a memory of deep relaxation that you can use to relax yourself. When you are relaxed, you cannot be angry, upset, anxious, afraid, frustrated, stressed, or in pain, because relaxation is the physical and emotional opposite of those feelings.*

*You can deepen your relaxation now (and when you do this exercise on your own), by counting slowly down from 20 to 1. With each number that you count, you will find yourself going deeper and deeper into relaxation and hypnosis. So right now, just read the numbers slowly, let yourself go,* and enjoy the experience of going deeper into relaxation and hypnosis. As you go deeper, you will feel better with each number that you read. 20, 19, 18, 17, 16, 15, 14, 13, 12, 11, 10, 9, 8, 7, 6, 5, 4, 3, 2, 1.

You are now learning how to do your own self-hypnosis. When you want to practice your own self-hypnosis and relaxation, you can do what you are reading here now, by yourself, without having to read anything. Ideally, that would be first thing in the morning before breakfast, and again late in the afternoon or some time before dinner, for about ten to fifteen minutes at each sitting. Find a comfortable chair to sit in, off by yourself. Your feet flat on the floor, with your hands palms down on your thighs. In order to visually focus your attention, instead of reading one group of words after another, as you are doing here, look at some object not too far away to fix your gaze, and pay attention to your breathing. Don't try to change your breathing.

Shortly, your eyelids will begin to feel heavier, just as you have experienced while reading this exercise, and you will also notice that your eyelids are blinking more frequently than usual. When you notice this, gently close your eyes and continue to pay attention to your breathing without trying to change your breathing. Your breathing will change all by itself. If you find your mind wandering, the moment you realize it is wandering, bring your attention back to your breathing and allow yourself to relax even more. You can also help yourself to go even deeper into relaxation and hypnosis by counting silently and slowly down from 20 to 1, just as you did here. With each number that you count to yourself, you go deeper and deeper into relaxation and hypnosis.

When your deepest mind is fully aware of how much comfort you have and knows it can maintain that comfort for some time after you awaken yourself from self-hypnosis, and knows it can continue to process what you have accomplished during your self-hypnosis, your eyelids will blink several times and then they will open, and you will emerge from hypnosis fully alert, sound in mind, body, and in control of your feelings and relaxed and comfortable. Now, when your deepest mind feels that these instructions for self-hypnosis are clear and locked in place in your subconscious, your eyelids will blink several times and then open wide, and you will emerge from this self-hypnosis feeling alert, relaxed and comfortable. How do you feel? How was that?

# ◎ Deepening Your Relaxation and Self-Hypnosis

When I use the term "deepen," as I did in the induction above, I am not referring to increasing distance traveled, but rather to increasing the *quality* of your self-hypnosis trance experience, that is, how comfortable you feel. You feel more relaxed and less relaxed at different times during your self-hypnosis trance experience. To deepen your self-hypnosis trance state means to help yourself into greater relaxation and comfort.

Going deeper also means helping yourself go further into your altered state, into your experience; to become more absorbed and more at ease. It means to get further into "the flow," become less distracted by extraneous environmental stimuli and more and more open to the relaxation experience. You feel more comfortable, and there is a further reduction in the mental chatter in your head. There is a further lessening of *trying* to relax.

The deeper you go, the greater your rapport with yourself. Your ability to use your imagination is heightened. You feel more calm and relaxed. Going deeper into self-hypnosis helps you get more comfortable and further out of pain. The quality of your self-hypnosis experience is heightened.

## Self-Hypnosis Method 3:
## Dr. Cheek's Pencil-Drop Method

This method was described by Dr. David Cheek (Cheek 1994). It combines both *visual* and *tactile-kinesthetic* sensory systems. It also adds an *auditory* component through counting down and the use of the cue word "relax." Dr. Cheek's method makes it possible to go very deeply into self-hypnosis and relaxation. Remember that you don't *have* to go very deep, but the deeper you do go, the more effectively you will reduce your discomfort.

Dr. Cheek pointed out that the altered state we call "hypnosis" can occur directly, when you sit back in a comfortable, balanced, and open position as I have instructed you to do. So situate yourself comfortably again now so that you can read yourself into self-hypnosis with the script below. As you did earlier, read slowly, silently or quietly aloud, a few words at a time, keeping your head as still as you comfortably can.

> *Hold a pen or pencil in one hand and prop that hand and forearm up on your elbow at a forty-five degree angle. Place the instrument between your thumb and index finger in such a way that it will easily drop onto*

*your lap, the floor, or onto your table or chair when your fingers pull apart. Your fingers will pull apart and drop the instrument when you are able to recall how numb and pins-and-needles–like your other arm would feel if you had been lying on it for a couple of hours while you were sleeping.*

*Now, as you continue to read each one of these words, bring up the image of a lighted candle of your favorite color and scented fragrance, sitting on a table about six feet in front of you. If you have trouble seeing it, just wait for the image to come up for you. Everyone knows what a candle flame looks like and how it behaves, and everyone is able to visualize at a subconscious level. Recall that the flame of a candle is always moving. It gets larger and smaller and swings a little from side to side with the gentle flow of air currents in the room.*

*While you are watching that candle flame in your mind's eye, gradually relax the muscles of your forehead, neck, and shoulders. These are the muscles we tend to tense up when we are scared or anxious or uncomfortable. As you relax them, you feel more calm and comfortable. Take a few moments to relax them now, and feel yourself relaxing more and more with each breath that you exhale.  Now, as you read the numbers from 20 down to 1 below, you relax even more with each number you read. Please think or say to yourself, "Relax," with each number you read. Okay. Begin reading the numbers now. 20, 19, 18, 17, 16, 15, 14, 13, 12, 11, 10, 9, 8, 7, 6, 5, 4, 3, 2, 1.*

*If your fingers are still holding the instrument, let it drop now, and on some level, you will get the message from your other arm and hand that they feel numb and pins-and-needles.  When your inner mind knows that you are feeling twice as relaxed as you were before, or that your arm is twice as numb, your index finger on the hand that was holding the pen or pencil will lift up all by itself to let you know. Just keep on relaxing more and more with each breath that you take and each word that you read and wait for your index finger to lift all by itself.*

*Each time you repeat this exercise your experience of self- hypnosis will be more comfortable. You will find that you are able to go deeper and experience the suggested changes in your experience more easily. This is an especially helpful self-hypnosis method for helping you become more comfortable.*

*When your deepest mind is fully aware of how much comfort you have now and knows it can maintain that comfort for some time after you awaken, your eyes will blink several times and you will emerge from your self-hypnosis and feel fully alert, sound in mind and body, in control of your feelings, and relaxed and comfortable. How do you feel? How was that?*

# ◎ Awakening or Alerting Methods

There are alternative ways to alert yourself or awaken yourself or "emerge," or come back out of self-hypnosis. The one I have been using with you communicates a "win-win" situation to your unconscious. That is, that you will alert when you agree to feel better, pure and simple, and not before! That is why I like it. I owe this alerting routine to Dabney Ewin, who first made me aware of it.

Another simple, alternative alerting method for bringing yourself out of self-hypnosis is to count yourself up from 1 to 5. You can give yourself these simple suggestions.

> *When you are ready to awaken from your self-hypnosis and bring your comfort and relaxation with you, count to yourself from 1 up to 5. When you say 5, you will feel wide awake and alert, but also very relaxed, calm, and comfortable at the same time. So, if you're ready to exit self-hypnosis now, you may begin counting. 1, 2, 3, 4, 5. Wide awake, alert and yet relaxed at the same time.*

## Self-Hypnosis Method 4:
## The Arm-Drop Method

The following self-hypnosis method is simple, brief, and easily learned. It is *visual* and *tactile-kinesthetic*. It takes advantage of several natural, physical phenomena, most notably gravity. This method is a popular induction and has been used in one form or another by various well-known hypnosis practitioners. I was instructed in the method by the late Helen Watkins, who was a clinical psychologist at the University of Montana in Missoula, a master clinical hypnosis practitioner and teacher, and the cofounder of Ego State Therapy. This is an adaptation of her version.

Read the script below several times first to get the steps of the method down and then close this book and do it now.

> *Put one hand or the other up in the air and concentrate on the finger of your choice. You can do this with your eyes open or your eyes closed, it makes no difference. If you decide to keep your eyes open, then stare at*

*your chosen finger. But if you decide to close your eyes, then stare at the finger in your imagination. Either way, you will find that the other fingers begin to fade away.*

*As you continue to concentrate on that finger, you will also find that the hand and arm become heavy, and that the more you concentrate on that finger, the heavier the hand and arm become. As the hand and arm begin to feel heavier, the hand begins to move down. As the hand and arm move down, you move down with it, into a comfortable state of relaxation. But you will not enter a deep state until the hand is all the way down and resting on your lap or belly, the arm rests if you are sitting in a chair, or the table, or the bed if you are lying down. When your hand is resting comfortably and you are in a deep state of self-hypnosis, pay attention to your breathing, and breathe in such a way that your abdomen moves in and out and your chest barely moves at all. Notice that every time you breathe out, you go down a little bit deeper, more and more relaxed with each breath you exhale. And the deeper you go, the better you feel. Every breath you exhale is taking you deeper into this relaxed state.*

*Now, as you keep on breathing deeply and easily, I'd like you to imagine a set of twenty stairs covered with a thick, plush carpet in your favorite color. Imagine you are standing at the top of the stairs and feeling the softness of the carpet beneath your feet, your feet just kind of easing and sinking into the carpet. On one side is a railing of highly polished wood. You can glide your hand along that railing if you wish as you walk down those stairs, counting each step that you take. And with every step that you take and count, go deeper and deeper into your relaxed state and feel more comfortable.*

*When you are at the bottom of the stairs, there's a door that you can open. When you open that door, you can enter your favorite "laughing place." Everyone has a laughing place where they feel really happy, content, pleased, comfortable, or actually feel like laughing. So, now you enter your favorite laughing place.*

*Just let yourself stay in your laughing place for a little while and enjoy being in this deeply relaxed state. You're building a memory of this relaxing experience that will continue. You will be able to borrow back this memory of comfortable relaxation to relax yourself whenever you want to. When you are ready to awaken yourself, you'll be able to do so by climbing back up those twenty steps, counting each step as you climb back up. When you reach the twentieth step, your eyes will open wide, and you'll feel wide awake, refreshed, alert, comfortable, and yet relaxed at the same time. The comfort you bring back with you will last for some time after you awaken from self-hypnosis.*

*From now on, you will be able to do your own self-relaxation in the same way that you just experienced it. That was nice and easy, wasn't it?*

*Here's a short list of laughing places to help you remember your own.*

» A snowy winter day in the woods in the mountains or a snowy winter day at the seashore

» A warm summer day in the woods or an autumn day in the woods

» Sunday at your favorite park

» A warm, crackling fireplace in a mountain cabin

» A sunny summer day at the beach

» Listening to the crickets in the forest on an August night

» A running stream in the forest or a secluded mountain waterfall

» The pitter patter of raindrops during a summer rain shower

» A warm bubble bath on a cold snowy winter day

» A Caribbean hideaway or sitting on a lounge under a thatched hut on a tropical beach

» A desert sunset or sunrise

» A desert mountain waterfall or spring

» Floating on a rubber raft in a mountain lake on a sunny summer day

» Floating on a rubber raft in a motel pool on a sunny summer day in the desert

» Sitting in the orchestra front row at the opera or at a Broadway play

» Praying at your church, synagogue, mosque, or other religious place of worship

» Sailing on the ocean or on a lake

» Walking in the woods or on the beach

» Engaging in your favorite hobby or sport

» A time and place in your life when you laughed a lot

» A very special, safe and pleasant, real or imagined experience from your childhood

» When you first fell in love for the first time

» Your favorite room in your house

» The aromas of cooking or baking in the kitchen

» The scent of a favorite person's perfume or cologne

» The sound of a loved one's voice

» A loved one's caress

» Your favorite scent, fragrance or aroma

» Your favorite piece of music or sound

» The most pleasant feeling you ever had or can imagine

## Self-Hypnosis Method 5:
## The Magnetic-Hands Method

The following is a visual and tactile-kinesthetic self-hypnosis induction method. It is one of my personal favorites because it involves paying attention to part of the energy system in your body. The steps are given below. As in earlier exercises, read each step, then do what it says. Then, read the next step, do that one, and so on. Work your way through the entire exercise in this manner. After you have practiced going through all of the steps several times and understand them, put this book down and do the method in one continuous flow.

*Sit comfortably, feet flat on the floor, back supported, and hands resting palms down on your thighs.*

Do this and then read the next step.

*Extend both arms out in front of you, slightly bent at the elbows, with your palms facing each other about eight to nine inches apart. Keep your fingers separated on each hand. Stare at the space between your hands. As you do so, also pay attention to your breathing without trying to change your breathing. Just let yourself breathe easily and normally. Don't hold your breath. Consider the suggestions you've just read, do what's instructed, experience the effects, and then read the next step.*

*Now feel the energy field in the space between and around your hands. That energy field is real and is pulling your hands toward each other. Can you feel that energy and your hands drawing together? Perhaps you can see the energy field, like an aura.*

Consider the suggestions you've just read, do what's instructed, experience the effects, and then read the next step.

*There is a magnetic field surrounding each hand and in between your hands. This energy field creates a magnetic force you can feel, and it is causing your hands to pull together. It is a manifestation of the universal life-force energy. The Chinese call it "ki" or "chi." The Indians call it "prana." Feel this magnetic energy field pulling your hands together. Concentrate on the feeling and keep breathing easily and normally. It is as if your hands are magnets and the opposite poles of these magnets are pulling together, drawing your hands together. It takes effort to keep your hands apart as you continue to concentrate on the space between your hands.*

Consider the suggestions you've just read, do what's instructed, experience the effects, then read on.

*As you continue to stare at and concentrate on the energy-filled space between your hands, you feel your hands pulling together. You also notice that your eyelids are blinking more frequently and are feeling heavier. Shortly, you may feel like closing your eyes, but don't close them until your hands come together. You'll notice how much more comfortable your eyes feel once you close them. When you do close your eyes, you will be sufficiently focused and absorbed, and you will enter self-hypnosis, but not before. When your hands begin to touch, position them so that the fingertips of one hand are touching the fingertips of your other hand.*

Consider these suggestions, do what's instructed, experience the effects, then read the next step.

*Pay attention to the pulsing you feel in your fingertips. Let that pulsing generate a feeling of warmth in your fingertips. Spread that warmth, that life-force energy, through your hands, into your arms, and up into your shoulders. Continue to pay attention to your breathing and breathe easily and normally. When you feel the warmth in your upper arms and shoulders, gently pull your hands apart and position your hands again with palms resting down on your thighs.*

Consider the suggestions you've just read, do what's instructed, experience the effects, then read the next step.

*Feel the energy and warmth in your hands. This is healing energy. Intend for that healing energy to flow through your body, and send that energy to where it's needed most. Feel grounded and strong as that healing energy circulates through your body, filling you with positive energy. Breathe normally and let that healing energy circulate with your breath throughout your body. Permit your inner mind to make the adjustments necessary to help you feel more comfortable.*

Consider the suggestions you've just read, do what's instructed, experience the effects, then read the last step.

*When your deepest mind is satisfied that it has sent enough healing energy to where it is most needed in your body, you can awaken. You will be fully aware of how much comfort you have now and your deepest mind will be satisfied that it can maintain your new comfort for some time after this session. Blink your eyes, open them wide, and come back fully alert, sound in mind, sound in body, and in control of your feelings.*

## Self-Hypnosis Method 6:
## The Eye-Roll Induction Method

This is a tactile-kinesthetic induction method originated by Dr. Herbert Spiegel (Spiegel and Spiegel 1978) and adapted by many others. My version is an adaptation of Dr. Spiegel's Eye-Roll Method and Dr. Ewin's Rapid Eye-Roll Induction (Ewin 1998). There are three basic steps. At the count of "one," you do *one* thing, at the count of "two," you do *two* things, and at the count of "three," you do *three* things. Then you deepen your relaxation experience through progressive muscle relaxation and active sensory imagination.

Read through my version below. After you've read my step-by-step instructions several times, and know what to do, practice the procedure without reading and experience how it feels.

*At "one," you do one thing. Roll your eyes up toward your eyebrows then all the way up toward the top of your head. At "two," as you continue looking upward with your eyes, you do two things. Take a deep breath and hold it while you let your eyelids slowly flutter down closed. At "three," keeping your eyelids closed and your eyes still looking upward, you do three things. Let that breath all the way out just like a balloon collapsing, relax your eyes, keeping your eyelids comfortably closed, and go more deeply relaxed than you've been in a long time. Eyes relaxed, jaws unclenched, shoulders droopy, arms limp, loose, and floppy, abdomen soft and relaxed, breathing calm and easy, legs loose and lazy, and your mind as relaxed as your body. Feeling calm, confident, peaceful, and safe.*

*Then, when you're ready, go to your favorite place in your mind and imagination. Experience the sights, sounds, words, music or songs, aromas, scents, tastes, pleasant feelings, any other people or living beings who might be around, the touch or caress of someone who loves you, and so on. All of these things make up your "laughing place."*

*When your inner mind knows you are so absorbed in your special, laughing place that nothing can bother or disturb you, let your index finger on your nondominant hand slowly lift up to verify that this is so. Then relax your index finger. When your inner mind is fully aware of how much comfort you have now and knows it can maintain this comfort for some time after you awaken from self-hypnosis, blink your eyes, open them wide and bring them back to focus, emerging from hypnosis fully alert, sound in mind, sound in body, and in control of your feelings.*

See how easy this method is? It's also brief and very portable. You can do it anywhere and anytime. Therefore, it's useful for instant relaxation whenever and wherever you need to relax instantly. If you're around people and don't want them to know you're doing it, you can camouflage it. This is how.

At "one," close your eyes and bring your hand up to your forehead as a signal to yourself that you're taking an instant relaxation break. It appears to others as if you're just rubbing your forehead and thinking to yourself. At "two," keeping your eyelids closed and your hand on your forehead, raise your eyes upward and take a deep breath and hold it. At "three," keeping your eyelids closed, relax your eyes, let that breath all the way out, and relax your entire body. Then think about and imagine being in your laughing place briefly, like you're taking a needed mini-vacation. When you're ready to return to normal awareness, blink your eyes and open them wide, remove your hand from your forehead, and resume being fully alert, sound in mind, sound in body, and in control of your feelings. That's all there is to it! That's easy, isn't it?

## Self-Hypnosis Method 7:
## The Relaxed Eyes and Counting Method

The following self-hypnosis induction method will help you reach a very deep level of relaxation quickly. It involves closing your eyes and, at first, focusing all of your attention on relaxing your eyes. Then, suggestions are made for spreading that relaxation through your body and deepening your relaxation through counting. This is a simple, effective, and quick hypnosis entry procedure that has been described in one form or another by several clinical hypnosis experts (Edmonston 1986; Elman 1964; Schafer 1996). Read the script below several times to get familiar with the procedure, and then do it.

*Comfortably situate yourself either in a sitting or reclining position. Close your eyes, and just sit or lie back and relax. Take a deep, deep breath and hold it for a few seconds. Then breathe out all the way and allow your eyes to completely relax. Let your eyelids remain closed and concentrate all of your attention on your eyes. Concentrate on relaxing the muscles around your eyes, more so and more so to the point where those eye muscles feel as if they won't work.*

*Allow yourself to experience your eyes as so very relaxed that they just want to remain closed, because they just do not feel like opening. When you feel that your eyes are so very relaxed that they just want to remain closed because they just do not feel like opening, spread that deep relaxation through your entire body. Let your body experience either a pleasant floating sensation, or just feel like it's sinking down into the chair or recliner or bed.*

*Now open your eyes briefly and repeat the procedure two times. By the third time, you'll have easily tripled your depth of relaxation. You'll feel the difference when you have gotten to this deep level of relaxation.*

*By now, you have attained deep physical relaxation. To get deep mental relaxation, begin counting slowly from 100 backwards. You can say the numbers softly to yourself or count silently in your head. Each time you say a number, you will feel as if your relaxation is doubling so that by the time you reach the number 90, if you even reach 90, you will feel so relaxed that it will seem as if there aren't any more numbers. It will feel as if the numbers have just disappeared, or it will feel like it's just too much effort to continue to keep track of the count. Start with the idea of making this happen, and it will happen—this is what you'll experience.*

*Once you've experienced this, just remain in deep relaxation until you are ready to emerge back into your normal waking state. While you remain in deep relaxation, you may enjoy just paying attention to your breathing without trying to change your breathing. Or you may enjoy just drifting or floating or hovering or staying absorbed in this engaged, neutral, joyful, open, and, yes, kind of altered state. And when you are ready to emerge or awaken yourself from your self-hypnosis, just count yourself back up from 1 to 5. At the count of 5, you'll feel alert, refreshed, renewed, restored, revitalized, and yet relaxed, calm, and comfortable at the same time. And your comfort will last for some time after you emerge from your self-hypnosis.*

That is all there is to it. Isn't that pleasant and easy?

## Self-Hypnosis Method 8:
## Absorption in Sounds

**A metronome.** Used for decades, a handy, inexpensive external aid to induce self-hypnosis is the metronome. This is a device that ticks off regular beats, and it is available in most musical instrument supply stores. It can be used to gently pace and guide yourself into a relaxed state because you can adjust the speed of the metronome's beat.

> As you listen to the beat of the metronome, the tapping or the clicking, you can feel yourself gradually becoming more and more relaxed. You may also find it interesting that as the beat slows down, you find yourself slowing down, relaxing more and more, gently shifting into a more relaxed and comfortable state of being in the moment. It's almost as if the beat of the little metronome paces the rhythm of your pulse, the pace of your breathing getting slower, more even, and more regular.

**Imagined and actual sounds.** You may wish to purchase a commercial tape or digital device so that you can play your favorite soothing sounds to help you relax and enter a self-hypnosis state. Alternatively, you can focus on select sounds in your imagination.

> Can you recall the natural soothing sounds of a flowing, babbling brook in the woods? Can you recall the sounds of ocean waves washing onto the beach? How about the pitter-patter of rain drops outside on the grass or on a patio during a summer rain on a humid summer day? Can you hear in your "mind's ear" the rushing sounds of a waterfall? How about the sounds in the forest or in the woods on a summer evening? What sounds do you find especially pleasant, calming, soothing, and relaxing? Take several quiet minutes and focus on imagining these sounds.

**Listening to music.** Listening to music is a great way to relax. Choose a piece of music on CD or tape that you are familiar with and that you find totally pleasing and relaxing. Put the music on, sit back and relax as you listen to it, and become totally absorbed in the musical progressions, the sounds and rhythms of the instruments, and the pleasant melodies.

**Use of a mantra.** The use of a mantra like those used in the Eastern meditation tradition can also be a helpful way of entering self-hypnosis and improving your ability to concentrate and direct your focus of attention. It simply involves choosing a word or brief phrase that is neutral, or that has a special, positive meaning. For ten to fifteen minutes, sit upright (so you won't fall asleep), spine erect, in a firm but comfortable chair, with your feet flat on the floor, and your hands on your thighs. Just think your chosen mantra word or phrase over and over again to yourself. Listen to it passively in your mind's ear as opposed to saying it actively.

Depending on what feels most comfortable for you, you can time the sound of the mantra to your breathing (for example, hearing it or repeating it silently each time you exhale), or you can just hear it in any rhythm or pattern that it takes on its own without any need to control it. When your mind wanders, as soon as you realize it is wandering, just bring your attention back to the sound of your mantra.

A type of Zen concentration meditation method is to focus your attention on a real or imagined repeating sound; for example, water falling or babbling, chimes, a ringing bell, a gong. Another concentration method that we have already described is to simply concentrate on your breathing without trying to change your breathing.

**Chanting and singing.** Chanting or singing can be a helpful way to enter relaxation. You may hum a tune or sound. Singing a song to yourself can be very pleasantly absorbing. Or, you can pick a hymn or psalm or chant with special significance and chant it quietly to yourself. It is your choice.

## ◎ Learning to Use Self-Hypnosis to Cope with Pain

I have devoted this chapter to describing alternative methods for entering and exiting self-hypnosis. Once you have experienced several different ways to enter a self-hypnosis trance and have chosen a method that appeals to you to practice, the next issue is what can you then *do* with self-hypnosis? How can you actually utilize self-hypnosis skills for coping with pain?

One answer to the question is to use self-hypnosis regularly to alter your state of consciousness and enter deep relaxation. That is a valid use. We have already talked about this. When you are relaxed, you cannot be tense, pressured, stressed, or in pain at the same time. The regular practice of self-relaxation through self-hypnosis recharges your batteries, so to speak. It replenishes and restores your energy reserves that have been drained by continued pain.

There is a growing body of evidence from the evolving field of psycho-neuro-immunology (the study of interrelationships between psychological and behavioral processes, neurological and hormonal processes, and the health of the immune system) that the regular practice of self-relaxation and controlled imagination is rejuvenating, renewing, restoring, revitalizing, and can strengthen your immune system. These effects can also improve your pain tolerance!

That is why you should take at least a week simply to practice inducing self-hypnosis for ten to fifteen minutes, twice a day. Use the induction method you favor to imprint the repeated healing experience of deep relaxation. This will start the process of positive change and prepare you for continuing the positive-change process.

In the chapters that follow, we shall explore different ways of employing self-hypnosis skills for coping with pain and changing your pain experience. You will see how easy it is to use hypnotic coping strategies and trance-state suggestions to change your pain experience and *hypnotize yourself out of pain now!* Because you have been able to choose your self-induction method, the method you have chosen will work for *you.* In the following chapters, you will continue to make choices, choosing different methods for helping yourself out of pain.

# FIVE

# Choose the Right Hypnotic Coping Strategy: Thinking and Behavioral Methods

*Self-hypnosis can be a safe and effective way to control or diminish chronic pain, as well as the negativity that often comes with it . . . Self-hypnosis can enable you to channel your ability to put your whole brain to work for you when you need it. The goal of hypnosis is for you to gain control.*

**—Devin Starlanyl and**

**Mary Ellen Copeland, M.S., M.A.**

Now that you know how to enter and exit self-hypnosis, it is best if you practice your chosen self-hypnosis method twice a day for about ten to fifteen minutes at each session. Your self-hypnosis practice sessions repeatedly imprint the healing experience of deep relaxation. After about a week of continuing this process faithfully, you can be confident that you have begun the process of positive change. At this point, you are ready to explore different ways of *employing* and *extending* your self-hypnosis skills to cope more comfortably with pain and change your pain experience.

Recall that the six D's of hypnotic coping are *deep relaxation, decatastrophizing, direction, distraction, distortion,* and *dissociation.* In this chapter, I will explain thinking and behavioral methods of coping. These include decatastrophizing and direction. In the next chapter, I will explain distraction and imagination methods, including distraction, distortion, and dissociation.

## ◎ How to Use the Next Three Chapters

Read through the explanatory material and exercises in this chapter and the next. This will familiarize you with the range of hypnotic coping strategies available. Become aware of which ones appeal to you and that you feel will work for you. Then proceed to chapter 7, where I will help you put it all together. In chapter 7, you will learn what you need to know about choosing, using, and formulating waking and trance-state suggestions. You will learn how to employ the thinking, behavioral, distraction, and imagination coping methods described in this chapter and the next both in a waking state and in self-hypnosis trance to imprint new resources in your unconscious. You will learn how to combine self-suggestions with self-hypnosis effectively to change your pain experience.

## ◎ Stay Focused

A self-suggestion is an idea that you give to yourself that can help you change the way you feel and think. For example, these are all self-suggestions: 1. After I read this chapter, I will understand how to change the way I think about my pain; 2. After I read this chapter, I will understand how to consistently exercise greater control over my behavior; and 3. After I read this chapter, I will feel more confident about using self-hypnosis to relieve my pain.

There are many self-suggestions provided in the following pages. In fact, for each of the six D's, I provide a separate list of additional self-suggestions to augment those given in the section devoted to that class of hypnotic coping strategies. Now, sometimes having too many choices is not a great thing. One can become overwhelmed with too many choices. However, I prefer to err, if I do, on the side of giving you more choices than you need, than too few choices. The point I want to make is the following one: Choose *one* to *three*, and never more than three, self-suggestions to work with at any given time. Work with the suggestions you have chosen repeatedly for a while *before* you switch to one to three different suggestions to work with.

If you proceed as I advise, when the time comes to work with self-suggestions, you will have ample choices, and you will stay focused. Consequently, the few suggestions that you choose to focus on will imprint in your unconscious, or they might not. If they do, that means they are right for you. If they do not, that means you need to choose one to three alternative self-suggestions to focus on and to work with.

# ◎ Deep Relaxation: The First D

The first D of pain coping is *deep relaxation*. We have already covered this D in detail in chapters 3 and 4. I need not say much more about it here because you already know how to do it. If you have read this far, you have experienced how easy and pleasant it is. You understand that deep relaxation does not need to be that "deep" to be pleasant, comforting, and healing.

Recall, as I stated earlier, that when I talk about trance depth, I'm referring to the *quality* of your self-hypnosis and relaxation experience. As I shall explain in specific step-by-step terms in chapter 7, you can use self-hypnosis to change your pain experience. You need not go deep into "la-la land" to do this.

### Some Additional "Deep Relaxation" Self-Suggestions

The list below provides you with choices of deep relaxation self-suggestions to augment and amplify your experience of deep relaxation. In chapter 7, we are going to explore in detail how to use self-suggestions. At this point, however, with deep relaxation as your main goal, simply choose two to three of the suggestions in the list below to read to yourself several times before you enter self-hypnosis from now on. Work with a few self-suggestions repeatedly for a while and then switch to several others. By working in this way, you will find it easy to remain focused.

1. My mind is quiet and still.

2. My body is calm and relaxed.

3. I am safe and at peace.

4. My body knows what it needs to do to make my muscles soft and comfortable. I can help by taking a deep breath, and as I exhale, just letting go.

5. I'm relaxing all of my muscles from the top of my head way down to the tips of my toes.

6. Every nerve and fiber in my body is loose, limp, and lazy.

7.  My arms and legs feel like those of a rag doll.

8.  My arms and legs feel like soft strands of overcooked spaghetti.

9.  I'm gradually relaxing the muscles of my forehead, face, neck, and shoulders.

10. With each breath I exhale, my muscles relax more and more.

11. As I count slowly from 10 down to 1, with each number, I relax more deeply.

12. I feel a wave of relaxation washing down my body, from my head to my toes.

13. Stress just drains away like water flowing out through a hole in the bottom of a glass.

14. With each normal breath that I take, I relax more and more.

15. I breathe in relaxation and breathe out tension and stress.

# ◎ Decatastrophizing: The Second D

When you believe that your discomfort will lead to the worst possible consequences and that the situation or your life will turn into a disaster, that is called *catastrophizing*. Catastrophizing, or extreme, negative, doom and gloom thinking intensifies your suffering, worsens your pain, and adds to your problems. It elevates the status of an uncomfortable experience from bad to worst.

Therefore, the second D of pain coping is *decatastrophizing*. It means dispelling the disaster from your experience of discomfort. It also means cutting the calamity or catastrophe out of your pain experience. Decatastrophizing suspends the suffering element from your pain and arrests your anguish.

Please understand that decatastrophizing is not a way to ignore reality or sugarcoat the badness of a difficult situation. It's a way to keep your thoughts, feelings, and reactions in check so that you can function and achieve your important goals. Our minds have a tendency to imagine calamities, catastrophes, and disasters when circumstances are adverse, but things usually aren't that bad. "Bad" does not equal "disastrous" or "awful."

Therefore, to cope effectively, you have to train yourself to control your mental activity. You cannot afford to let your negative thoughts and feelings get away from you and get out of hand. You must tame your thoughts in order to tame your pain.

The Chinese have an ancient proverb that says that a crisis is really an opportunity in disguise. When you decatastrophize, you transform a potential crisis in your mind into an opportunity to see options and alternatives for coping more effectively with the situation. You also alleviate or avoid unnecessary suffering by neutralizing excessive negativity and deescalating the intensity or extremity of your response.

**Decatastrophizing and the Brain.** Recall our earlier discussion in chapter 1 of the neurology of pain? Decatastrophizing works from the top down. It is initiated in the highest levels of the brain, its central control center, which is the frontal and prefrontal cortex. This part of the brain is the seat of the conscious mind. It has connections to nerve fiber pathways that transmit information to and from the deepest, innermost parts of the brain, called the subcortex. The sub-cortex is one of the seats of your inner mind or unconscious.

There are areas deep inside your brain, in your subcortex, that control your emotional reactions as well as your physiological drives, such as hunger and thirst. Deep within your brain's subcortex there also resides a central relay station where physical sensations, including pain, are initially processed when they first reach the brain. This relay station is called the *thalamus.*

Once physical sensations are identified and processed in the thalamus, their sensory signals are routed and dispatched. The thalamus is like a central mail room. As with the mail, not every message passes through intact all the way up to your brain's central processing and control center. Some messages are intercepted, held back, or inhibited. Others are damaged, dampened, or distorted. Still others do pass through intact, and some are actually accentuated, amplified, and sent through as overnight, express mail.

The subcortical areas deep inside your brain are connected in turn to the base of your brain, or your brain stem. Your brain stem controls all of your essential physiological functions that keep you alive (breathing, heartbeat, blood pressure, alertness, sleeping, basic reflexes).

Decatastrophizing thought processes begin in your brain's frontal and pre-frontal cortex, the seat of your executive control functions. This is the part of your brain that makes you distinctly human. It enables you to plan, organize, and execute your behaviors, symbolize, represent, and recall information, and interpret your experience. When you choose to decatastrophize, your brain sends messages from your frontal and prefrontal cortex down the pathways described above. This somehow results in closing the pain gate in your spinal cord.

**Waking State Decatastrophizing.** You don't need to be in self-hypnosis trance to decatastrophize. In fact, when you first learn how to decatastrophize, you should practice it in the waking state. Later on, after you gain experience, you can decatastrophize in or out of self-hypnosis trance. Disputation (explained below), which is one method of decatastrophizing, is a conscious waking state procedure. On the other hand, reframing (explained below), which is another method, is both a conscious and unconscious process.

**Disputation.** Disputation is one method of decatastrophizing. *Disputation* means challenging your negative, unhelpful thoughts, and changing them. This technique is done in the waking state because you need to be aware consciously of what it is that you need to challenge and change. It is a rational, logical procedure.

When you catch a negative thought that is making you feel bad, you need to let go of that stress-producing thought. One way is to interrupt the thought and redirect your attention to something else that is neutral, such as your breathing. Another way is to challenge or dispute the thought. When you realize that the thought is not true, you can cancel the thought, and replace it with a functional, stress-reducing thought. This is done in the waking state. With repetition and practice, however, disputation does tend to become automatic and unconscious.

**Disputation Case Example.** As an example of disputation, you might consider John, a thirty-eight-year-old engineer who was a patient of mine with chronic low-back pain. He wanted to know why he was unable to be as logical and rational in coping with his pain as he was in his work and also in helping other people deal with their problems. In four sessions of psychotherapy, I helped John to develop the habit of recognizing when he was thinking or dwelling on negative, catastrophic thoughts, and to pinpoint those thoughts. I taught him to pick out one or two of his most negative thoughts and to write them down. He stated that "somehow or other, just seeing them on paper seems to take the lie out of them!" By writing his negative thoughts down, he trained himself to see how fantastic and unlikely many of them really were.

I also taught John to ask himself several logical questions to challenge his negative thoughts. For example: "Is it possible that I'm blowing things up out of proportion? Is there any valid evidence that this will happen to me? What evidence is there? How do I know? Am I letting my fears get away from me and out of hand? Am I letting my fears rule me now? How likely is this to happen? What is a more reasonable thing to expect?"

## Exercise 5.1: Self-Analysis

Take a few minutes to reflect on the following questions. Write your responses in your notebook.

How often do you catastrophize? Can you recall any recent situations when you felt very depressed or anxious about your pain? Can you recall what you were thinking at the time? What were you most afraid of happening? Can you identify specific negative, malignant, or toxic thoughts? Did any of these thoughts blow things out of proportion? In what ways? Did you allow your worst fears to take over? Did things end up as bad as you had feared? Can you "put the lie" to these thoughts now and dispute them? If you had done this *then*, how would your experience have changed?

### *Reframing*

The most important coping tool that you always have available to you is reframing. *Reframing* means changing the way you think about something without necessarily changing that something (Zarren and Eimer 2001). It means changing the meaning of your beliefs that continue to produce dysfunctional behavior and experiences. This may not change the substance of the problem, but it does change the way you think about yourself in relation to the problem.

To decatastrophize or cut the calamity or catastrophe out of an unfortunate experience and arrest your anguish, you must *reframe* the experience. Changing the way you think about your pain, reframing it, provides the basis for taking constructive action, as opposed to continuing to have destructive reactions.

For example, continuing to think that your pain is fixed, permanent, constant, unpredictable, uncontrollable, and mysterious is likely to foster continuing feelings of helplessness and hopelessness. How do you cope when you feel that nothing you do makes any difference? The answer is that you tend to be passive and reactive as opposed to being active and proactive. Rather than seeing options and alternatives, you see only more suffering.

If you believe that there is a vicious pain loop in your central nervous system and that there is nothing you can do to break the circle then you're not likely to do much. If you perceive your pain to be an unyielding medium of torture and your life to be a torture chamber with no escape hatch, then what is there left to do but continue to suffer? However, what if you were willing to consider the possibility that your pain is not all bad—that it has something to teach you? That it could offer a very valuable lesson you might as well try to learn since you've already paid for it ("pained" for it) many times over? This would open up different possibilities, would it not?

Everything that happens happens for a reason, although we might not yet know what that reason is. If everything that can be done and should be done for your pain has been done, and there is no reason for it to continue, but it does continue, then there must be a reason. Much could be gained by discovering the reason. There is usually a physical reason that cannot be fixed or corrected. If this is so, one lesson to be learned is how to accept this fact and deal with it. Another lesson to be learned is how you can lessen the pain's impact on you. Still another lesson to learn concerns how you can improve the quality of your life despite the burden of pain that you have.

## Exercise 5.2: Exploring and Reframing the Pain's Meaning

Take a few minutes to reflect on the following questions. Write your responses in your notebook.

Everything has meaning. What does your pain mean to you? Does your pain mean to tell you that you need to modify your lifestyle? Soften up? Harden up? Get stronger? Become more tolerant? Be more forgiving? Less angry? Less reactive? More compassionate, caring, or empathic? Take better care of yourself? Learn to appreciate your life more and take the good things in life less for granted?

Does your pain mean to tell you that you need to realize and accept that you're not the same as you once were? You have something important to teach others to help them cope better with the adversities in their lives? Is it time to start being more empathic? Start enjoying all of the little pleasures in life? Start appreciating the goodness in people? Start learning how to say thank you?

I had kept an old painting from my childhood. It must have been in its dusty, faded, worn old wooden frame for over fifty years. One day, I decided to change that frame. So I had the painting reframed. When my mother came to visit, she didn't recognize that painting. She asked me if I had bought the interesting new painting at the picture shop in the mall!

If you accept the view that your brain has the ability to slow down or reduce the traffic on the "pain highway" in your spinal cord, then you will be open to different possibilities for controlling the traffic. If you believe that your spinal cord is like a bundle of telecommunications cables and your brain is the central control center, then you will be open to different possibilities for rerouting the messages, slowing them down, blocking, intercepting, or masking them, and so on. In order to avoid invasive interventions (like attempting to redirect or halt the traffic on the highway, your spinal cord, itself) you'll need to work on the central control center, your brain.

Reframing is a more general, broad-based, and flexible coping tool than disputation. Disputation is very logical and orderly because it involves rationally reevaluating your thinking about your pain and your situation. Reframing, on the other hand, need not be logical or orderly. Reframing, in fact, frequently can be super-charged by good doses of imagination and creativity, as I have just demonstrated.

Reframing is crucial for countering helplessness and hopelessness. When you feel helpless and hopeless, your problems feel unsolvable and your situation feels like a disaster or a catastrophe. The pathway out of such despair is to reframe the problematic situation; to put a new frame on an old situation. Applied to your pain management, the idea is to train yourself to change how you think about your pain, the meaning of your pain, yourself, your purpose, and what you can do to cope. Reframing enables you to neutralize and replace negative thoughts or beliefs that make your pain problem feel insurmountable, as if an impassable wall blocks your path to freedom from pain.

## Exercise 5.3: A Path In the Woods

Imagine yourself walking down a beautiful country path through the woods. The path leads to a beautiful lake further on where you very much want to go and relax. Suddenly, you come upon a very high stone wall that cuts right across the path and into the woods on both sides of the path. You are completely blocked from proceeding further unless you can somehow get over or through that solid stone wall. You try climbing it, but you can't. You try pushing against it, but it doesn't budge. As your frustration grows, your attempts become more frantic, and you may even bloody your hands in the process of trying so hard. How can you get to the other side of the wall? More of the same is certainly not the answer. And yet, all too often, we do more of the same even though it is not effective, hoping that increasing the effort will work. But it doesn't.

You need to recognize that there are other choices, other options, that can be applied to solving your problem. Pushing against an immovable stone wall harder and harder still will not move the wall. However, backing off and rethinking possible solutions to the problem may produce better results.

You can calmly look to the right and left of the path, near the wall, for a pathway you can follow that may take you to a door or to the end of the wall. This makes more sense. You do so, and you notice a small clearing and path on your right near the wall. You follow it and are joyfully relieved to see an unlocked gate through the wall to the other side. There you see a lovely flower-covered meadow leading to that serene lake on the other side. The solution to the problem was not to push so hard doing the same thing that didn't work, but to recognize that you have choices and to make a different choice. (Zarren and Eimer 2001, 33)

Reframing is a way of changing the belief that you are trapped to the belief that you have choices. It can involve changing the meaning of any of the following: beliefs, attitudes, habit patterns, negative or destructive labels, feelings, or behaviors, and helps to open the way for positive emotional and behavioral change. The way you think about something can be changed even though "the facts" may remain the same. The original situation may in fact remain unchanged, but you can perceive the situation from a new point of view. What is changed, as a result of reframing, is the meaning you give to the situation. This change in meaning *can* change the consequences of the situation, although its concrete facts may remain unchanged, at least initially.

**A Reframing Case Example.** Christine was a registered nurse who had been put on "light duty" at the hospital where she worked after sustaining a back injury lifting a patient. The incident happened five months before her referral to me. When I saw Christine for an initial evaluation, she was sullen and angry. She felt she was permanently injured and would never be the same again. She described her pain as starting in her low back and shooting down her right leg. The pain was "constant, gnawing, pressing, pinching, shooting, and burning." She was on heavy doses of opioid painkillers, which made her feel more irritable, depressed, and drowsy.

We reviewed her story from the present backward to the time of her injury while she was in hypnosis, and she revealed that one of the doctors who was prescribing her pain medicine made the remark that she would "have to learn to live with the pain." At the time of that visit, she was very emotionally distraught and in a very impressionable state. My further questioning revealed that her unconscious mind had literally interpreted the doctor's statement to mean that, *if she lost the pain, she would die.* Therefore, the implication was that she needed to hold on to the pain to survive.

This imprinted negative belief was keeping her from getting better and had to be reframed. To not reframe this blocking belief and proceed with any form of pain management would be like trying to break through a stone wall. I told her that the doctor had certainly not intended to give her that message, but that he was not an expert on using the right language to communicate with the unconscious, so he chose the wrong words while she was in a very impressionable state of mind. I told her that he probably meant to say: "You're acting as if you're an emotional wreck. You need to get yourself together now, start dealing with your situation better, and get on with your life." This reframed her dysfunctional belief that if she gave up the pain she would die into the functional belief that she needed to give up her pain so that she could resume living her life.

### Negative Emotional Overlay

Negative, dysfunctional thoughts like the one Christine suffered under make persistent pain worse by creating a negative emotional overlay on top of the physical pain. This increases your emotional distress and suffering and hoists up the "hurt level" of your pain—how much you actually *feel* your pain. Therefore, it is helpful to catch such thoughts and then dispute or reframe them. This can lift off the negative emotional overlay.

# Exercise 5.4: The ABC's of Decatastrophizing

The following exercise will help you practice asking yourself the right self-analysis questions to decatastrophize a stressful or painful situation and lift off the negative emotional overlay. These questions guide you in examining your thinking so that you can catch your "thinking errors" (negative, unhelpful thoughts), correct them, and begin feeling better. Record your responses to this exercise in your notebook.

Begin by dividing a blank sheet of paper into three columns. Going from left to right, label the columns "A," "B," and "C." Think of a situation that is upsetting, aggravating, irritating, depressing, threatening, or painful. We will refer to this situation as the (A)ctivating Event. Ask yourself what is happening or has happened that's upsetting to you (for example, a worsening of your pain, an argument with your spouse, being treated rudely or unfairly, hearing bad news, etc.). Write down the essential facts of this (A)ctivating Event in the column you labeled "A."

Next, ask yourself how and what you are, or were, feeling emotionally (for example, depressed, anxious, scared, angry, etc.). Write your responses in the C column labeled "C." Also, identify any associated physical sensations (for example, more pain, sweating, lump in the throat, heavy chest, shaky, dizzy, etc.). Write them down in the C column also. Label this material the "Emotional and Physical (C)onsequences" of the situation, or the "C's."

The emotional and physical Consequences (the C's) of the Activating event (the A) are associated with how you are interpreting the situation—that is, your thoughts about the situation—or what you are thinking. Therefore, the next step is to identify and write down in the B column your thoughts and beliefs about the situation. Asking yourself the following questions will help you uncover your negative and stress-producing thoughts.

1.    What went through (is going through) my mind?  What was I (am I) thinking?

2.    What was I (am I) telling myself? What do I believe about this situation?

3.    What thoughts, beliefs, images, memories, daydreams, or recollections led to these unpleasant feelings?

Write down what comes up for you in the middle, B column. Label your answers to the above questions your "(B)eliefs," or your "B's." See, it's as simple as A, B, and C!

Now you are ready to ask yourself some of the following questions in order to challenge, question, and dispute your negative stress-producing thoughts and beliefs (your B's), the conclusions you drew about the situation. Do this on a separate page.

1.  What does this situation mean to me (or about me)? Is there another way to look at it?

2.  How do I know this is true? Where's the evidence?

3.  Is there another explanation? Is there another way to look at this situation?

4.  What if it is true? What would that mean to me? So then what? What would that mean?

5.  What is the worst that could happen? Play it out in my mind to the end. And then what? What is the likelihood of it happening?

6.  If this were to happen, what of it? How much would it really matter?

7.  What are the "advantages and disadvantages" of thinking and acting and feeling like this?

8.  How might this situation be used to my advantage? What can I learn from this?

9.  Is my thinking realistic? If it isn't, how isn't it?


The next fourteen questions will ask about any exaggerations, errors, or distortions in your thinking that may be holding you back.


1.  Am I thinking in *all or nothing* terms?

2.  Am I assuming I can *read someone's mind*, that I know what they're thinking or how they feel without them telling me? Do I have a crystal ball that can enable me to predict the future?

3.  Am I letting myself get overly emotional? Am I taking this too personally? Am I letting my feelings rule me? Am I putting the cart before the horse?

4.  Am I jumping to unwarranted conclusions? Am I assuming something without having enough evidence? Am I thinking rationally?

5.  Am I blowing things way out of proportion?

6.  Am I overgeneralizing?

7. Am I setting up unfair expectations or standards? Am I making an unfair comparison?

8. Am I disqualifying any positives? Am I being too much of a perfectionist?

9. Am I looking at the glass as *half full* or *half empty*?

10. Am I possibly projecting blame unfairly onto either myself or someone else?

11. Am I basing my entire self-worth on one or two things?

12. Am I expecting too much?

13. Am I erroneously assuming that the world must be fair, or that things mustn't be the way they are?

14. Am I expecting magic or a miracle?

The next group of questions will lead you to begin thinking about what coping possibilities you can use now or may want to try.

1. What can I tell myself to help me cope and get through this?

2. What images can I picture or thoughts can I think to make me feel better?

3. Can I mentally rehearse a more positive, desirable outcome?

4. Who is talking inside of me? Whose voice is it?

5. How bad or uncomfortable do I feel on a scale of 1 to 10 or 1 to 100?

6. What would I tell someone else who was going through the same thing?

7. How might I *distract* myself from the pain?

8. What can I direct myself to *do* or *think* to lessen the pain and make me more comfortable?

After you have gone through this process, you will have come up with other ways of thinking about the situation or event that are more functional and stress-reducing. After you have gone through this process several times with different situations, the new, more positive thoughts you come up with will provide you with material for constructing specific suggestions to give yourself in self-hypnosis. In chapter 7, I will explain how to build appropriate self-suggestions and use them with self-hypnosis. After you have gone through this decatastrophizing and disputation process enough times, it will become easier and more and more automatic.

## Taming Your Thinking

By now, hopefully you realize that one of the key coping tools for "taming" persistent pain is "taming" your thinking processes. Taming your thinking processes largely involves getting into the habit of consciously and subconsciously responding to your internal chatter in a constructive manner. Decatastrophizing, including reframing and disputation, are a great way for you to "talk back" to your unhelpful thoughts.

Your mind is always active. So, you can't stop thoughts from automatically popping into your head in the first place. But you need not let an unproductive or destructive thought stream continue without adding your constructive and corrective conscious input. You have the ability to *respond* to your thoughts, so you can do something about them. This gives you choices in terms of how you respond to your pain.

One choice is to just do nothing and let the thought stream continue. Another choice is to try to ignore unwanted thoughts, or turn them off. You can also shout silently in your head, "Stop those thoughts now!" You can divert or redirect your attention elsewhere to take your mind off of the unwanted thoughts. You can also interrupt the thought stream, for instance by taking several slow, deep breaths, and then go on to do something else.

You can also respond to the thoughts directly with the intent of changing them by using the strategies I explained above. Remember: Just because you have a thought does not mean that it is a valid thought, or that it accurately reflects reality. Also, you are *not* your thoughts!

## Sometimes Doing Nothing Is Best

Sometimes doing nothing is the best choice, if it is a conscious one. I myself am a very goal-oriented person. Therefore, I hate the fact that my physical condition often limits what I can do, how much I can do, and when I can do it. My pain often has a mind of its own. Sometimes, it just takes too much energy that I don't have to exercise, or work, or write, etc. At such times, I have a choice. One choice is to bitch and moan and groan and get angry or depressed. Another choice is to make a *conscious choice* to listen to my body. My body may be asking me to rest, to stop, and just do nothing for a while.

If I choose to listen and do nothing for a while, it is a conscious choice. It's also different from being controlled by my pain. This is different from rewarding myself for giving in to my pain or rewarding my pain for acting up by stopping what I'm doing and taking some "downtime."

If, when I am hurting and feeling drained, I choose to listen to my body and do nothing for a while, I really am doing something. I have reframed the situation so that instead of interpreting it in terms of being controlled or victimized by the pain, I experience it as an opportunity to take a break in order to recharge my internal batteries. This is empowering as opposed to restraining because it enables me to cut through the energy drain and reduce the strain of the pain.

## Some Additional Decatastrophizing Self-Suggestions

The list below provides you with choices of decatastrophizing self-suggestions to help you in reframing your pain. As I instructed you to do earlier with the deep relaxation self-suggestions, simply choose *two* or *three* of the suggestions in the list below to read to yourself several times before you enter self-hypnosis from now on. If you choose at this point to work with decatatrophizing, focus on these and put aside the deep relaxation self-suggestions that you may have been working with up until now. The guiding principle is to work with a few self-suggestions repeatedly for a while, and then switch to others. By working in this way, you will find it easy to remain focused, and you will succeed in imprinting the suggestions you choose in your unconscious.

1. I have strong coping skills that help me deal effectively with the pain.

2. I need not accept every thought or feeling as valid.

3. I catch negative, stress-producing thoughts and eliminate them.

4. I interrupt negative, stress-producing thoughts and feelings.

5. I question and challenge negative, stress-producing thoughts.

6. I replace stress-producing thoughts with stress-reducing thoughts that help me cope better.

7. I am in charge.

8. It may feel unpleasant or uncomfortable, but it does not have to feel painful.

9.   I no longer need to automatically interpret discomfort as meaning harm.

10.   I can manage this pain. I can handle this.

11.   I optimize the control I do have in managing the discomfort.

12.   I can tolerate this and more.

13.   I can stand the pain.

14.   I've survived worse, so I can cope with this.

15.   I need no longer suffer.

16.   I can still enjoy things.

17.   Whenever I feel stressed, I accept the feelings and stay calm.

18.   No pain lasts forever. This is a temporary problem. It won't last.

19.   Pure pain without suffering does not hurt as much.

20.   It's only pain!

21.   I am *not* my thoughts!

# ◎ Direction: The Third D

The third D of pain coping is *direction*. "Direction" refers to the act or process of controlling, guiding, governing, instructing, or supervising your thoughts and actions. It involves setting goals to achieve and then behaving in a way that leads to the achievement of those goals. Self-hypnosis coping skills help you direct or guide your thoughts and behaviors in line with your positive and healthy intentions.

Applied to your own coping, direction means controlling your own behaviors and thoughts to *maximize* short-term and long-term pleasure and well-being and *minimize* short-term and long-term pain. It involves instructing yourself to think and behave in a functional way in your day-to-day life. It includes using "positive self-talk" and "positive **Self-suggestion.**" These two tools entail saying positive affirmations to yourself, preparing yourself to handle difficult, uncomfortable, or painful situations, talking yourself through those situations, and giving yourself direct suggestions for desired changes in your experience.

### Stress Inoculation Training or SIT

Stress Inoculation Training or "SIT" is a direction strategy in which you employ self-statements or "self-talk" to control or instruct your thinking and behavior just *before, during,* and *after* a bad episode of pain. It is a structured coping plan for making your experience more tolerable and controllable. It can also be called "self-instructional training." SIT should be practiced and rehearsed so that it becomes second nature.

SIT enables you to be your own coach, an energetic and encouraging coach to guide and cheerlead you on. It is one of the strategies that sports psychologists employ in coaching athletes to improve their game. Industrial and organizational psychologists also employ SIT with corporate executives to coach them to be more productive in business. Here are the fundamentals of SIT applied to pain management.

There are fours steps to the process: 1. Picking up on early cues that tell you it is time to prepare for a rise in discomfort; 2. Coping with a pain episode after it has started up; 3. Dealing with the pain at its worst, and keeping yourself together when it's at its maximum strength, and 4. Settling back down after it's all over, rewarding yourself, and giving yourself credit for handling the pain episode successfully.

## Exercise 5.5:  Stress Inoculation Training

When you rehearse the steps of SIT in a waking state or in self-hypnosis, you are imprinting a "mind-set" in both your conscious and unconscious mind. It is a mind-set that prepares you for dealing with your pain when it gets so bad that it really challenges the limits of your mental and physical tolerance. Please use your notebook to write down your responses in the following exercise.

1.  **Prepare yourself.** As soon as you notice that the pain is beginning to increase, you can get prepared, or "psyched," to deal with it by telling yourself things such as:

    *I'm now going to get ready to deal with this. I can handle this. I have coped with this before. This time it will be easier for me to manage. I will be okay. I can listen to what my body is telling me. I can learn something from this. It's a shame to waste "good pain."*

    What else might you tell yourself?

2.  **Begin to cope.** As the pain begins to get stronger, you too can get stronger as you tell yourself things such as:

*I'm doing fine. I will not let the pain get the best of me. There are plenty of things that I can do to make this tolerable. I can do my deep breathing. I can just notice the sensations. I can shift my attention elsewhere. I can do my instant relaxation. I can go into self-hypnosis. I can think of something funny. I can filter the hurt out of the pain. I can make comforting pictures in my mind.*

What else might you tell yourself at this point?

3. **Handling the worst moments.** When the pain is at its worst, you can be at your strongest. You can remind yourself of the following:

*This is a temporary problem. No pain lasts forever. I am handling this. I will continue to breathe comfortably. I can stand this. I can get through this. I can remain strong. I am my own best friend. I can continue to coach myself through this. This pain, too, shall pass. I will only have as much pain as necessary. I will not let negative thinking get the better of me. Keep talking to myself. I can stick with the task. Just notice the sensations while I breathe through them.*

What else might you tell yourself at these most difficult moments?

4. **Self-reinforcement.** When the pain flare-up begins to subside, you can remember to give yourself credit for coping and staying in control. You can tell yourself things like:

*I did it! I remained strong. I coped well. I stuck to my plan. I used my coping skills well. I can feel good about myself. I deserve to give myself credit or a pat on the back for sticking with the plan under fire. It will be easier next time. How nice that I now have a coping plan in place.*

What else might you tell yourself to help you feel better about yourself and your coping ability? After you get into the habit of doing this, in what ways do you think you will feel different?

## Pain Behaviors and Well Behaviors

Given that nobody is perfect, we all engage in behaviors that we would like to do less of, either because the behaviors are dysfunctional or just because we do too much of them (like drinking or eating too much, working out physically too hard, working too many hours, sleeping too much, etc.). These are termed "behavioral excesses." In addition, we all have things that we would like to start doing that we are not doing currently, as well as things we would like to do more of. These can be termed "behavioral deficits" (like starting to exercise, sleeping more, eating regularly, working fixed hours, controlling our temper, etc.).

We can set limited goals for ourselves to start doing one thing that we are not doing, or diminish our doing of something that we need to cut down on. This can help us begin to establish new, healthy habit patterns. Establishing healthy habits is especially important for people who have the added burden in life of having to cope with a chronic illness or chronic pain. It is a necessity if you want to lead some semblance of an orderly life.

Healthy habits help you to conserve precious energy. There are certain behavioral coaching principles that can help you to establish and maintain healthy habits. Being aware of and following these principles can also help you create and maintain more order and discipline in your daily life. This will help you restore more control over your life and your pain. Shortly, I will outline twelve behavioral coaching principles that are in your own best interest to follow.

**Pain Behaviors.** "Pain behaviors" refer to those behaviors that reinforce your pain and increase the dysfunction in your day-to-day life. In contrast, the term "well behaviors" refers to adaptive, functional behaviors that are associated with diminished pain and disability and increased functionality. Both pain behaviors and well behaviors can be overt and observable by others, or covert and invisible to others.

**Overt Pain Behaviors.** Things like limping, grimacing, moaning, groaning, repeatedly rubbing parts of your body that hurt, muscle guarding and bracing, stiffening, avoiding movement, pacing, shaking, frequent sighing, screaming, and crying are overt pain behaviors. Others include: complaining a lot about your pain, making statements communicating hopelessness, helplessness, depression, anger, fear, anxiety, or other forms of distress and suffering, and making excessive requests for assistance. Frequent downtime behaviors, such as lying down often, sleeping a lot, avoiding most activities, and withdrawing from social contact, are also overt pain behaviors.

**Covert Pain Behaviors.** These are internal behaviors and therefore are not directly observable to others. This category would include such things as: habitual negative thinking; constantly feeling depressed, anxious, fearful, or angry; having repeated morbid images and daydreams (for example, having intrusive visions of yourself being helpless, in agony, becoming worse, etc.); sustaining a loss of motivation to do things; and being excessively preoccupied with your discomfort and pain sensations.

**Well Behaviors.** In contrast, healthy "well behaviors" are functional thoughts, feelings, and behavioral responses to pain that are not ruled by pain. This category of adaptive behaviors includes such things as following an activity schedule, doing your self-hypnosis and self-relaxation, using the power of positive self-suggestion, and employing functional coping skills. Other functional well behaviors, along with pertinent self-suggestions, include:

1.  Using pain medicine (that is prescribed by only one physician—the one who is treating your pain) on a regular dosing schedule so that you have steady blood levels of the medicine and it is always in your system.

    **Self-suggestion.** *I keep a steady level of pain medicine in my system so that I stay comfortable and continuously get enough pain relief.*

2.  Going to sleep at the same time every night and getting up at the same time every morning. Limiting your bed to only two things: sleeping and sex.

    **Self-suggestion.** *When I lay my head down on my pillow in bed at the same time every night, I get the best night's sleep and the rest that I need. When I awaken at the same time every morning, I feel rested, refreshed, and ready to get up.*

3.  Exercising regularly, based on a predetermined and realistic quota that's geared to your level of conditioning, rather than on how you feel at the moment or on your momentary pain tolerance.

    **Self-suggestion.** *I get the most from my workouts when I plan them. So, I decide beforehand how long and how hard I'm going to exercise.*

Thinking positively, and interrupting and challenging your negative thought stream, fall into the category of covert well behaviors. These behaviors are internal (not readily observable by others), functional, learnable, and trainable, as we have already discussed. These behaviors, in turn, affect other covert or internal responses, such as your emotional states (feeling confident as opposed to feeling nervous, fearful, or insecure; calm as opposed to angry; hopeful as opposed to depressed), and your physiology (feeling relaxed as opposed to nervous, tense, stressed, etc.).

## Twelve Behavioral-Coaching Principles

As promised, here are the twelve principles that will help you adopt more healthful behaviors.

**Mental rehearsal.** What's the best psychological way to counter fatigue *instantly*? The answer is mental rehearsal to activate dormant or temporarily inactive "action potentials" (firing capabilities of the sensory and motor nerves that innervate or excite the sensory receptors and muscle fibers involved in adaptive behaviors) (Evans 2001). So when you are feeling too tired to engage in an activity you want or need to engage in now (such as getting out of bed), visualize yourself doing that activity (like getting out of bed) for thirty to sixty seconds before actually doing it. Visualize using all of your preferred sensory systems (your active sensory imagination). See, feel, and hear (and if relevant, smell and taste) yourself engaging in the activity. This is a technique that actually is borrowed from sports psychology.

For example, to drum up the momentum to get out of bed in the morning, I usually spend about a minute seeing, feeling, and hearing myself getting out of bed and getting started with my initial morning activities. I imagine smelling and tasting the freshly brewed, strong coffee. I imagine feeling the comforting tactile-kinesthetic stimulation of my warm shower. I imagine the relief I feel when my back is stretched out and warmed up.

While I employ my active sensory imagination, I also pay attention to my breathing without trying to change my breathing. However, sometimes I intentionally will breathe in a slow, deep, regular, and controlled manner. My immediate goal is to stimulate mental and physical action potentials (nerve cell firing capabilities) to help me overcome the stiffness and sluggishness I always feel when I wake up every morning.

**Positive reinforcement.** Enhance your motivation to engage in an unpleasant, nonreinforcing activity that is good for you (such as exercise or eating your vegetables) by rewarding yourself after you do it with something that is very pleasant for you. For example, if you love to eat ice cream (unless you are allergic to ice cream, and then choose something else that you like), give yourself ice cream as a reward after you do your prescribed back exercises. That's positive reinforcement. But remember also to positively reinforce yourself internally for doing the right thing. Praise yourself. Give yourself a "pat on the back." If you can't reach your back (pun intended), just tell yourself that you've done well.

**Self-suggestion.** *When I give myself credit for taking good care of myself, this positively increases my energy and my comfort.*

**Take baby steps.** Don't bite off more than you can chew all at once. That's a sure recipe for re-injury whether you're dealing with working in the garden, or sitting at the computer, or exercising. Take small steps. Each step moves you closer and closer to your goal. But set realistic and reasonable goals. Be patient with yourself.

Patience is the ability to wait calmly for something desired. Patience is a virtue, and virtue is its own reward. Pace yourself. You may just have to acknowledge and bring yourself to accept that, since your injury, you are not the same person you once were, and that you may never be capable of doing what you used to do.

**Self-suggestion.** *When I'm patient with myself and others, I'm able to achieve my goals comfortably.*

**Be flexible and conserve.** Plan your days and your week, but be flexible (in more ways than one). You may have to alter your plans. Learn to tolerate uncertainty; after all, nobody can predict the future. Learn to tolerate the frustration of not always finishing an important task. You can do the rest tomorrow and are more likely to be able to do so if you are comfortable. When energy is in short supply, it's important to conserve it.

**Self-suggestion.** *I conserve my energy and comfort by staying mentally flexible.*

**Get away from pain.** Set realistic quotas on what you do. Try to divorce your activities from pain so that you are not controlled by it.

**Self-suggestion.** *I plan what I intend to accomplish ahead of time so that I conserve my energy and my comfort.*

**Be persistent.** When you have persistent pain, perseverance, determination, resolve, and persistence are good qualities to have. They help you keep going when you would rather lay down in bed. It is understandable if you feel like giving up at times. But you need not! However, don't be like that battery bunny on TV. Don't keep going and going and going and going. You will run out of energy. Remember to pace yourself.

**Self-suggestion.** *I am as determined and persistent as my pain and more so.*

**Seek the middle ground.** Train your significant others (spouse, children, parents, friends) to neither overcater to you and do too much for you, or be punitive and blaming with you. Neither situation is functional. The most functional situation is the middle ground. Train your significant others to be understanding, but do not allow them to become enablers of your dysfunction. Try to accept as little help with your basic activities of daily living as possible. But remember flexibility. Don't be afraid to ask for help when you need it. Remember that no one can ever feel your pain. Don't punish people around you for not being able to totally understand!

> **Self-suggestion.** *I accept my responsibility to stay as functional as I can, but I am willing to ask others for help when it is appropriate.*

**Stop doing pain behaviors.** We went through a pretty exhaustive list of pain behaviors earlier. Pain behaviors breed further dysfunction and more grief, pain, and suffering. So, develop the habit of catching yourself when you're doing pain behaviors and simply stop doing them. Then reward yourself for doing so.

> **Self-suggestion.** *My unconscious notifies me when I'm doing a pain behavior, and I consciously interrupt it, back off, and do something different.*

**Counter your deconditioning.** If necessary, work with a physical therapist who understands chronic pain and your particular medical condition. People with chronic pain have the unfortunate tendency to get out of shape and become deconditioned because exercise often hurts. Unfortunately, the more deconditioned a person becomes, the more pain-prone the person becomes also.

So, it is important to prevent or work to undo or *counter* deconditioning. Also, exercise, especially aerobic exercise, such as walking, helps the body to release its own internal opioid-like chemicals, which are called endorphins and enkephalins. These natural products can help with your pain. Thus, it is important to exercise as much as possible, keeping your own particular physical limitations and condition in mind. Your body has a limitless supply of these pain-relieving chemicals. Physical exercise in moderation and doing thing you enjoy helps your body unlock and release these chemicals.

> **Self-suggestion.** *When I exercise regularly and appropriately, I increase my energy, my strength, my flexibility, my mental alertness, and my comfort.*

**Learn assertiveness and make it a habit.** *Assertiveness,* as opposed to aggressiveness or hostility, can be defined as the ability to stand up for yourself in an argument, defend your interests and position, and protect your rights without losing control. Assertiveness means being able to say no, make your preferences and decisions clear about matters of direct concern to you, and express your feelings or disagreement in a clear and appropriate manner. It also involves being able to set limits and make choices about what you will do or not do in an interpersonal relationship.

Many people lack skills that would allow them to do these things. It is important to develop such skills. It simply makes good sense and takes just a little courage to start standing up for yourself without becoming hostile or aggressive. Practicing your assertiveness skills can make them become second nature. Becoming more assertive can help you feel more in control and better able to get your needs met.

> **Self-suggestion.** *I stand up for myself because if I don't, nobody else will. I feel better when I assert my rights.*

**Avoid unfair comparisons.** You are unique. There is nobody else exactly like you in the entire world. Avoid comparing yourself to others, or at least catch yourself when you are doing it and stop it. I promise you that this will help you avoid needless grief. It is true that there are commonalities amongst humans because we are all human. And there are typically even more commonalities within different groups of humans (like for people with chronic pain within the same cultural, ethnic, or religious group). However, in truth, everyone's individual circumstances are unique.

Therefore, it isn't helpful to waste your precious energy on making unfair and probably invalid comparisons between yourself and others. Since no two people are alike, it just doesn't make sense to compare yourself to others. If you come up short, you end up feeling depressed, angry, or jealous, and these are self-defeating emotions.

> **Self-suggestion.** *I feel better and cope better when I accept the fact that I am a unique individual. There is no one else exactly like me in the whole wide world. Therefore, I need not compare myself to others.*

**Embrace self-acceptance.** You have as much intrinsic self-worth as the next person. You are no less worthy as a person, as a human being, than is the Queen of England or the President of the United States! By the same token, you are no more worthy as a person than the beggar on the street corner. Your self-worth as a *person* is a given. You are worthy because you are alive.

You can rate your skills and accomplishments, but it is invalid to rate your whole being. That is, in effect, what you do when you rate your self-worth. You deserve to do everything you can to live as comfortably as you can—you have suffered enough. Remember, pain may be mandatory, but suffering is optional. Let the suffering stop here! Accept your self fully with all of your imperfections and your pain.

> **Self-suggestion.** *I fully and completely accept myself even with all of my imperfections, my conditions, and my pain.*

## Striving Toward the Principles

As you know, these twelve points are principles, ideals to reach for and strive toward. As ideals, they are not going to be a snap to adopt. Admittedly, some principles are harder to follow than others. There are many shades of gray. So, what to do? I think the best solution is to be easy on yourself. Don't try to be perfect, even in following and living according to these principles. You have your whole lifetime to practice!

## Some Additional "Direction" Self-Suggestions

The list below provides you with choices of "direction" self-suggestions to help you take charge of your well behaviors. As I instructed you to do earlier with the decatastrophizing and deep relaxation self-suggestions, simply choose *two* or *three* of the suggestions in the list below to read to yourself several times before you enter self-hypnosis from now on. If you choose at this point to work with direction, focus on these behaviorally oriented self-suggestions and put aside the previous self-suggestions that you may have been working with up until now. Remember the guiding principle: Work with a few self-suggestions repeatedly for a while and then switch to several others. By working in this way, you will find it easy to remain focused, and you will succeed in imprinting the suggestions you choose in your unconscious.

1.  I act functionally, even when I feel uncomfortable. Other people need not know how or what I am feeling.

2.  I control the discomfort by using my head and orienting to my heart.

3.  I fully accept myself even though I still have this discomfort.

4. From this moment on, I am easier on myself and more forgiving.

5. I take satisfaction every day in handling my problems better and better.

6. Every day I find that the pain concerns me less and less and doesn't disturb me as much.

7. Easy does it. I am mastering my pain a little bit at a time.

8. I control my behavior and my thoughts for my own good.

9. I talk to myself positively.

10. I do good things for myself.

11. I make comforting pictures in my mind to diminish the discomfort.

12. I rid my mind of unwanted thoughts and retain positive and helpful thoughts.

13. I feel less angry, less needy, and more happy, peaceful, and content.

14. I have more self-confidence and greater self-esteem.

15. I have more control over my emotions and my behavior.

16. I am learning to get along with and befriend my pain.

17. The pain is just one part of me. I'm learning to relate to it and understand it. I am not my pain.

18. I stop and listen to what my body is telling me.

19. I'm doing the best I can to take better care of myself every day, from the time I get up in the morning to the time I go to sleep at night. I am not my pain.

20. Whenever I make a mistake, I realize I can correct that mistake by backing off and starting over or fixing what I have broken. Then I feel better.

21. I let go of unrealistic expectations about my pain, work, other people, and myself.

22. I have everything I need within myself to enjoy every minute of every day.

23. I expect things to turn out for the best when I act functionally.

24. I no longer need to feel that much discomfort.

25. I can step back and just watch what is going on.

26.   Whenever I feel uncomfortable, I take time to relax.

27.   I am going into self-hypnosis and relaxation for x minutes for the purpose of allowing my unconscious to make the adjustments necessary to help me feel [name your goals].

28.   When I awaken from my self-hypnosis, I feel wide awake, alert, refreshed, relaxed, and comfortable for some time after awakening.

29.   When I emerge from my self-hypnosis, I feel relaxed and prepared to sleep restfully throughout the night.

30.   When I awaken from my self-hypnosis, I feel motivated and full of energy.

# SIX

## Choose the Right Hypnotic Coping Strategy: Distraction and Imagination Methods

*One can always forget pain.*

**—Milton H. Erickson, M.D.**

## ◎ Distraction: The Fourth D

*Distraction* refers to diverting or redirecting your attention away from one thing toward another; for example, away from pain and toward something neutral, pleasant, or less uncomfortable.

Distraction is an effective pain-control strategy because the conscious mind can only process a finite or limited amount of input and information at one time. The unconscious, on the other hand, can process many things at the same time. So the goal in using the strategy of distraction is to introduce stimuli and sensations that compete with the pain sensations for your conscious attention. If these competing sensations get to your brain first, they can prevent the pain sensations from ever reaching your brain. They can at the least slow down the transmission of the pain sensations up your spinal cord.

### Distraction Works from the Bottom Up

When your conscious mind is paying attention to the sensations created by your rubbing or massaging the area of your body that hurts, it has less capacity to pay attention to pain sensations. Recall from our discussion of the neurology of pain in chapter 1 that the nerve fibers that transmit sensations of pressure, touch, and vibration carry information to the brain faster than those nerve fibers that transmit pain sensations. So, when the faster fibers are fired up through the introduction of tactile-kinesthetic stimulation such as touch, pressure, rubbing, or massage to the area of discomfort, their sensory signals get to the brain before the pain messages do. This tends to close the pain gate in the spinal cord.

Similarly, when your conscious mind is deeply absorbed in other tactile-kinesthetic activities such as paying attention to your breathing, enjoying the beach, writing, or painting, it cannot pay as much attention to pain. This also closes the pain gate.

Distraction is probably the easiest and simplest pain-coping strategy. It also capitalizes on the fact that what is most important at any given moment is what tends to capture your conscious attention. For example, if you were thinking about your pain and suddenly you heard a series of loud booms signalling the beginning of a thunderstorm, you would be likely to forget about your pain temporarily if you had forgotten to close the windows on your sun porch. You would most likely be redirecting your immediate attention to getting those windows closed before the porch got soaked!

In sum, distraction works by introducing stimulation that competes with the pain in your nervous system. The distractors generate competing nerve signals that beat the pain to the brain. They get there first and close the gate on pain.

**Case example.** The following example illustrates the mind-body-pain connection. When I take a walk, I usually get a deep gnawing pain in the muscles of my lower back. At the end of my walk, sometimes that pain is almost biting in its intensity. The application of ice usually helps to alleviate the pain by numbing the area, but little else helps. While I'm walking, if the pain gets really bad, my posture is affected. The pain causes my spine and back to list or tilt to one side. If I'm tired, and I don't have enough energy to compensate posturally for that tilt, this bows me over even more and further increases the pain.

One thing I discovered that helps is when I have a walking partner. If I become pleasantly distracted in conversation, I am temporarily less aware of the pain. Somehow or other, when I am less aware consciously of the pain, my spine does not seem to list quite as much. In this case, when the walk is over, I'm usually in not quite as much pain.

## Some Distraction Exercises

Distraction is easy. You just redirect your attention away from your discomfort and onto something else that is neutral, interesting, compelling, captivating, or engaging. You can do it in the waking state or in self-hypnosis. Below I provide a number of exercises that incorporate the strategy of distraction.

Do each of these exercises and discover which methods feel like they could make a difference and help you feel more comfortable. Familiarize yourself with all of the techniques so that you can find the methods that appeal to you and feel right.

Do a few exercises in a single practice session. A practice session doesn't need to last more than thirty minutes. You can work up to fifty minutes, which is the amount of time of a typical psychotherapy session in which hypnosis is used. If you want to work longer, you may, but don't try to do all of the exercises in one session. It's just too much.

Because you can choose the coping methods that are right for you, the methods you choose will work. After each exercise, write your responses down in your notebook. As with the self-hypnosis induction exercises in chapter 4, these exercises build on skills you have practiced earlier. See how easy it is?

It's perfectly all right if you choose to induce self-hypnosis before you do the following exercises. It is also perfectly okay if you choose to do the exercises in a normal, waking state. It's your choice. Either way is fine. Whether you choose to enter self-hypnosis first or do the exercises in a normal waking state, you are going to learn some important things based on your experience. You're going to learn which hypnotic coping strategies appeal to you, which ones feel right for you, and which ones do not.

After each exercise, there is a self-suggestion that conveys the essence of that hypnotic coping strategy. In chapter 7, I'll teach you how to employ the strategies you've discovered are right for you to change your pain experience on the deepest level that's possible for you. You'll be referring back to the self-suggestions for the strategies you choose to use.

In the future, you will be able to refer back to the hypnotic coping strategy exercises that are right for you before you do your self-hypnosis. In chapter 7, I'll also explain how to select, formulate, and use self-suggestions with and without self-hypnosis. After reading that chapter, when you go back to these hypnotic coping strategy exercises, you will have another choice you can make. You can either use the provided self-suggestion summarizing that coping strategy, or you can formulate your own special self-suggestions to give yourself for changing your pain experience before inducing self-hypnosis.

## Exercise 6.1: Fingers Rubbing Together

As described by Spiegel and Spiegel (1978), this tactile-kinesthetic method can be used whenever you begin to feel the discomfort rising. It enables you to filter your perception of the pain and concentrate on something else, whatever you choose.

First notice your level of pain. Then concentrate on one of your hands. Rub the fingers of that hand against each other and focus on the unique sensations that you can feel in those fingers. As you do this, describe to yourself the texture, temperature, and sensations that you feel. Now notice your pain level. Has it changed? This sequence of behaviors serves as a focusing mechanism. Rubbing your fingers together can also serve as a cue to take several deep breaths and remind yourself of something other than the pain.

**Self-suggestion.** *Concentrate on the engaging sensations of my fingers rubbing together.*

## Exercise 6.2: A Little Pain That Distracts

Again, notice your level of pain. Next, pinch the webbing between your thumb and index finger on one hand or with the other. Notice the force of your pinching. Does this help you become less aware of the other discomfort? Now increase the force of your pinching. Notice at what point you become noticeably less aware of the other discomfort.

**Self-suggestion.** *The stronger I pinch the webbing between my thumb and index finger, the less aware I become of the other discomfort.*

## Exercise 6.3: Therapeutic Touch and Self-Massage

Begin by noticing your level of discomfort. Now gently rub the area that hurts. Massage the skin and the muscles. This self-massage distracts your nervous system from the pain. As you do this, also intend that healing energy to flow through your hand into the area. Your body knows what to do to send healing energy to where it's needed. Pay attention to the point that you become noticeably less aware of the original discomfort.

Next, more vigorously rub and massage another area of your body that is distant from the area that hurts. Massage the skin and the muscles. This self-massage also distracts your nervous system from the pain. As you do this, also direct healing energy to flow through your hand and through your body into the area that needs more comfort. Your body knows what to do. Again, notice when you become less uncomfortable. In the back of your mind, think to yourself:

> **Self-suggestion.** As I massage myself, I am channeling into my body positive healing energy that flows to where it is needed most, and that increases my comfort and diminishes my discomfort.

## Exercise 6.4: Mindful Breathing

Pure pain doesn't hurt as much when you take away the fear of future pain and the upset over past pain. By taking a few minutes to just pay attention to your breathing without trying to change your breathing, just experiencing the sensations of your breath, you stay in the present and temporarily block out upsetting thoughts and feelings about the past or the future. So take a few minutes to do this now. Pay attention to your breathing, and help yourself stay focused by picking something interesting to look at that is not too far way. And as you continue to pay attention to your breathing, notice how your breathing changes all by itself. Do you also notice that you're feeling more relaxed? What effect does this have on your discomfort?

If you notice your mind wandering, just gently escort your mind back to your breathing and your visual attention back to the interesting something you have chosen to look at. As you practice this technique of "mindful breathing," you'll find that you become much more aware of each moment in the present. When you stay focused in the present, you cannot be upset by thoughts and feelings about the past or future. You become more mindful of how you feel in the present, at this very moment. Less mental and physical energy is spent worrying about future pain, or regretting or reliving past pain.

As you become more mindful of the present moment, you find that you begin to feel more in control because you're taking charge of how you employ your mental and emotional energy. So, whenever you catch yourself getting caught up in upsetting thoughts or becoming preoccupied with feelings of discomfort, you can now interrupt those thoughts and shift your attention to something else that is pleasant or neutral, such as your breathing, or a pleasant or interesting visual object. Then you're better able to leave any discomfort behind.

As you become more able to be in the present, you get better at interrupting negative, unproductive, or upsetting thoughts and thinking of something else. You realize that your thoughts, emotions, even your impulses are not reality. You create your own reality and are in charge of that reality. You are in charge of how you respond to what happens to you and around you.

**Self-suggestion.** *I can interrupt unpleasant thoughts and feelings by focusing my attention on my breathing. As I focus on my breathing and an interesting visual object, I shift into neutral.*

## Exercise 6.5: Slow, Deep Breathing

Another *kinesthetic* method is to take several very slow, deep breaths. Inhale slowly and deeply through your nose, breathing in relaxation, and exhale slowly through your mouth, breathing out tension and stress. Pay attention to the sensations of breathing slowly and deeply as you do this. Focus on the rising and falling of your chest or abdomen or the flow of air in through your nose and out through your mouth. What effect does this have on your comfort level?

**Self-suggestion.** *I can interrupt unpleasant thoughts and feelings by breathing slowly and deeply.*

## Exercise 6.6: Clenched Fist Technique

This is another *tactile-kinesthetic* method. Pay attention to the concentration of tension as you make a fist with one hand and squeeze it tighter and tighter. Keep squeezing it tighter. Now open your fist and feel the tension releasing. Shake your hand and release the rest of the tension. Keep shaking it. Can you make this procedure more effective by breathing in deeply as you clench your fist and exhaling slowly through your mouth as you unclench the fist? Does this help you release more tension?

**Self-suggestion.** *I squeeze all of my tension into my fist, and then relax my hand and release all of that tension.*

## Exercise 6.7: Focus on Sensations Elsewhere in Your Body

Can you notice where in your body you feel comfortable? In what ways do you feel comfortable in those parts of your body? Can you become more aware of any other parts of your body that have more comfortable sensations? Pay attention to where in your body you feel most comfortable. Also notice the many different sensations in your body; in your fingers, hands, arms, shoulders, neck, head, face, eyes, mouth, belly, back, buttocks, legs, feet, and so on. You can pay attention to lots of signals from your body, some from the pain area and others from different parts of your body that naturally feel comfortable. And with each and every breath you take, feel more comfortable. Imagine what it would feel like to be floating, to feel tingling, to be more relaxed, to feel warmer or cooler, and to be more comfortable. Find the most comfortable part of your body to pay attention to and the most comfortable position to assume. What other sensations do you notice in your body?

**Self-suggestion.** *I become aware of other parts of my body where I feel comfortable sensations.*

## Exercise 6.8: Pay Attention to Something Else

Can you temporarily pay attention to something else that is more comfortable or pleasant or neutral? Can you think about a really pleasant place where you would like to be right now? A happy or laughing place where you feel like laughing? Permit yourself to become absorbed in a pleasant memory and temporarily leave the discomfort behind. How was that?

**Self-suggestion.** *I can bring to mind and become deeply absorbed in a pleasant memory.*

## Exercise 6.9: Going with the Flow of Your Attention

What can you temporarily focus your attention on in your immediate physical surroundings? Can you study the grains in the wooden furniture? Can you study the different shades and colors in the wood? Can you visually trace the shape of the tiles in the bathroom or on the floor and study how they fit together? How many tiles are there in each row? Do you notice the shadows on the wall, or on the floor? Remove your shoes and rub your feet on the floor. Notice the feel of the carpet, hardwood floor, tiles, or linoleum. Listen to the sounds around you. What do you hear?

**Self-suggestion.** *I notice things all around me to which I can temporarily direct all of my attention.*

## Exercise 6.10:  Stream of Consciousness

Spend about five minutes simply following the train of thoughts in your stream of consciousness. Your mind is always active. Thoughts automatically come and go. You need not try to think anything deliberately or change anything. Just passively notice what comes and what goes. You need not try to prolong any thought, or stay with it any longer than it stays on its own. Just let it pass and be replaced by another thought.

> **Self-suggestion.** *Follow the train of thoughts in my stream of consciousness.*

## Exercise 6.11:  Mental Arithmetic

Do some mental arithmetic in your head. Perhaps you can count backwards from 200 by threes. Or, take the number two to the nth power. Or, count backwards from 500. Or, beginning with any number, keep adding five. Does this help you become less aware of the discomfort temporarily?

> **Self-suggestion.** *When I do mental arithmetic, all of my attention capacity is taken up, and it leaves no room in my conscious mind to notice anything else.*

## Exercise 6.12:  Become Absorbed in a Book or Movie

Become temporarily absorbed in a book, watching television, watching a movie, or listening to a piece of music. You can also simply imagine that you are doing so. Does this help you become less aware of the discomfort temporarily?

## Exercise 6.13:  Squeeze a Marble

The following *visual* and *tactile-kinesthetic* coping method is derived from Zarren's Marble Method, which was described in chapter 4 (page 59).
Use your marble to relax yourself, in seconds, whenever you need to most, wherever you are, without closing your eyes and without anyone knowing you are doing it. Just hold the marble in your hand, look at it, and roll it around. This will bring back an almost instant feeling of relaxation.  You can also squeeze the marble. The harder you squeeze it, the more comfortable you will feel. This is because, by squeezing your marble, you transfer some of the discomfort out of your body and into the marble. When you squeeze your marble, you concentrate all of your tension in your hand and let it go into

the marble. Your marble is very strong. It can absorb an unlimited amount of tension and discomfort. Just squeeze the strain and pain into the marble. It's a very valuable tool. You can use it to deal with stress or discomfort no matter when or where they may occur. If you don't have your marble with you, you can actively imagine holding it in your hand. Actively imagining your marble works just as well.

> **Self-suggestion.** *When I squeeze my marble, I transfer discomfort out of my body into the marble.*

## Self-Hypnosis Is a Distractor

Please be aware that when you employ any of the self-hypnosis induction methods described in chapter 4, you're distracting yourself from discomfort. Entering and exiting self-hypnosis removes you from the pain. Once you've chosen any self-hypnosis method that works well for you, it's possible to create an almost instant alert or waking version of your chosen method to relax yourself in seconds, whenever you need to, wherever you are, without anyone knowing you're doing it. The use of the marble for instant relaxation is one example.

Another example is taking several slow deep breaths while you focus your visual attention on some object not too far away. Another example is paying attention to your breathing without trying to change your breathing, with or without focusing your visual attention on some object not too far away at the same time. Still another example is the Eye-Roll Induction Technique described in chapter 4. Experiment with each of these methods. Which ones work best for you? Write your responses in your notebook.

# ◎ Distortion: The Fifth D

*Distortion* is a hypnotic coping strategy that involves re-interpreting the pain sensations so that you experience them as if they are something else. This involves changing, recoloring, and transforming your perception of pain sensations. For obvious reasons, this can be a very useful thing to do with pain sensations that are unnecessary remnants of a long-term physical condition you're well aware of and that is being medically treated. When your pain no longer serves a useful signalling function, you can turn down or change the signal and filter the hurt out of the pain (Spiegel and Spiegel 1978).

**Distortion Works from Both Ends.** Distortion works both from the bottom up and the top down neurologically. That is because it incorporates both distraction and re-interpretation (also called reframing). Distortion combines shifting your attention away from the pain to something else (distraction) with changing your interpretation of the pain (re-interpretation).

As you've read, distraction involves refocusing or shifting your attention to alternative stimulation that competes with the pain stimulation, and thus, blocks the pain signals on their way up the spinal cord to the brain. Re-interpretation or reframing involves changing the way you think about the pain sensations. This sends new and different messages from the brain down the spinal cord to the place in the back of the spinal cord where the pain transmitting nerve fibers interact. Both distraction and reframing contribute to closing the pain gate.

**The Components of Distortion.** The hypnotic strategy of distortion incorporates new sensory input (the distracting stimulus) and changes how the brain interprets the original sensory input (the pain). The bottom line is that distortion changes or transforms the pain sensations into something else—other, less painful sensations.

Distortion requires you to be able to do three things: 1. shift your attention, 2. become absorbed in your new object of attention, and 3. employ your active sensory imagination to create different sensory perceptions and impressions. Everyone can distract themselves from pain temporarily. Once you've distracted yourself, you move on to distort and transform the pain.

Following are the three steps to distortion.

1.  First, you shift your attention to different sensations, thoughts, or feelings. As I stated above, these can be stimuli unrelated to the pain or an element or facet of the pain sensations themselves.

2.  Second, you let these sensations, thoughts, or feelings become the generator of less uncomfortable (or more comfortable) countersensations that oppose the pain.

3.  Third, you let yourself become absorbed in these countersensations and employ your active sensory imagination to shape and develop them into a *changing* experience that's more comfortable and easier to handle.

### Some Distortion Exercises

When you *distort* your pain you *transform* it into something else that is less uncomfortable and more tolerable. Distortion takes a little practice. That's okay. The idea is to find a strategy or several strategies that are right for you and keep practicing them! As with distraction, you can distort your pain in the waking state or in self- hypnosis. I provide a number of exercises below for you to use.

Follow the same instructions that I gave you before for using the exercises in distraction. As before, do each of these exercises and discover which methods feel like they could make a positive difference for you. Find the methods that appeal to you and that feel right. Once again, because you can choose the coping methods that are right for you, the methods you choose will work. After each exercise, write your responses down in your notebook.

## Exercise 6.14: Reject Unnecessary Pain

Take several slow, deep breaths and concentrate on the pain. Get close to the pain and look at it, listen to it, and feel it. Study the sensations and imagine all of the electrical nerve fiber connections between the place where you feel the pain and your brain. Think of all of the nerve signals traveling up and down your spinal column between the area of the pain sensations and your brain. Let your nondominant index finger slowly rise all by itself when your inner mind has brought this information or picture to your conscious awareness. Then relax the finger.

Now, let your inner mind tell you just how much of that pain is necessary. Perhaps none of it is necessary anymore because it's already served its function, and the pain that is left is functionless. Or perhaps only some of it is necessary, and the rest is functionless, so that you need not keep all of it. When your inner mind informs you about how much pain needs to be retained to serve pain's protective function, your index finger on your nondominant hand will slowly rise all by itself. Then relax the finger. What have you learned? Write it down in your notebook now or after you complete this exercise.

Now that you have learned that all of the pain is no longer needed, instruct your inner mind to let go of the pain that's no longer needed. You can do this. Send away the pain that's no longer needed. Tell it to go away. If you have to, lead it out of your body. Now notice how you are feeling. Please rate your level of comfort now. What was this experience like?

**Self-suggestion.** *I am sending away the pain that's no longer needed. I am telling it to go away.*

## Exercise 6.15: The Flow and Discard Technique

Take a slow, deep breath, breathing in relaxation as you inhale through your nose, holding the breath for a few seconds, and then breathing out tension and stress through your mouth. Now inhale a second deep breath and make a tight fist with each hand. Hold this breath and clench your fists tighter and tighter. Feel the tension as you hold your breath and clench your fists. Now let your breath all the way out just like a balloon collapsing and relax your hands. Feel the release of tension.

Breathe normally. Now imagine your pain in the form of a substance that would permit it to flow; for example, as a syrupy, dark colored fluid. Then take a third slow, deep breath, clench your fists, and imagine that you're drawing up this substance into your arms and legs as you inhale. Hold your breath and visualize this substance. Then let your breath all the way out, relax your hands, and visualize this substance flowing down your arms into your hands and down your legs into your feet. Visualize this substance flowing out your fingertips, into the air and out your toes, into the ground. (Watch where you are standing or sitting if you don't want to stain your floor or carpet!) Take another deep breath and repeat the process. Then breathe normally again.

Now shake your hands vigorously and visualize the substance of the pain being released from your fingertips as little oily droplets into the air or as particles of lint being shaken free as you scatter them into the air. Can you visualize this and experience this? How was that? How did it feel? Do you feel more comfortable?

> **Self-suggestion.** *With the power of my mind, I discard unnecessary pain by inducing it to flow out of my body.*

## Exercise 6.16: The Floating and Temperature Technique

This exercise involves imagining that you're floating in water. For individuals who don't like water, the ways in which you can float comfortably are only limited by your imagination. For example, you can float on a cloud, on a comfortable mattress, in bed, on a magic carpet, in a zero-gravity chamber, in a protective bubble, in a hot-air balloon, in space, etc. You can enhance the pleasure of your floating experience by adjusting the temperature of your floating environment; making it warm and comfortable, or cool and comfortable.

Imagine that you are floating. Make the feeling of floating more vivid by imagining that you are floating in water. Let your inner mind decide whether to make it ice water or warm water. Your inner mind will choose either cold and comfortable or warm and comfortable depending on what your body needs. If your inner mind chooses ice water, as the water gets colder and colder you begin to feel a tingling icy numbness coming from the icy cold. This tingling numbness creates a protective shield around the pain area that filters the hurt out of the pain.

If your inner mind chooses warm water, as the water gets warmer and warmer you begin to feel the comforting, therapeutic, moist heat penetrating into the pain area. This causes more blood to flow into the area and filters the hurt out of the pain. How was that? What was that like?

> **Self-suggestion.** *By floating in the way I find most comfortable, I am filtering the hurt out of the pain.*

## Exercise 6.17: Spreading Pleasant Sensations

Imagine that you're floating in a way in which you feel safe and comfortable; for example, in a pool, a lake, a large bathtub, a large hot tub, on a cloud, a magic carpet, or on a water bed. Feel deeper and more relaxed with every breath. Each time you exhale, you let a little more tension out of your body. While you remain in this state of pleasant absorption, notice how your body is feeling. Are you comfortable? Is this pleasant? Do you enjoy the sensation of floating? Can you notice feeling pleasantly tingly anywhere? Where do you feel this pleasant tingling? Spend as much time as you need to notice where you feel tingling sensations in your body.

Now allow the pleasant tingling that you feel in your body to spread. Spread the pleasant tingling into your legs, into your arms, up and down your spine and back, and into your buttocks. And just imagine that it's a pleasant sense of either warm or cool tingling numbness, whichever feels better for you. It's penetrating deeper and deeper into your body so that you feel a pleasant sense of warm or cool tingling numbness, whatever feels better for you, spreading throughout your body and into and through the part of your body that needs to feel more comfortable.

You can imagine that this tingling is a kind of coolness, like you feel when you rub or apply ice on a part of your body. Or you can imagine that this tingling is a kind of moist warmth, like you feel when you apply a moist hot pack on a part of your body, or like when you take a warm shower, or a warm aromatic bubble bath, or like when you sit in a warm hot tub or in a whirlpool bath. Concentrate on the tingling and on a sense of cool tingling numbness or warm wet tingling sensations. Even though you're aware that the pain may be there, you can focus on this pleasant sense of floating throughout your body along with the cool, tingling numbness or warm wet tingling, to filter the hurt out of the pain.

Write in your notebook how this exercise in relaxed easy concentration, floating and tingling, felt.

> **Self-suggestion.** *I am focusing on spreading a sense of cool tingling numbness or warm wet tingling through my body and into the area that needs to feel more comfortable. This filters the hurt out of the pain.*

## Exercise 6.18: Comfort Transfer Techniques

The following exercises make use of the association between two generators of healing energy and the transformation or displacement of pain sensations and the transfer of comfort sensations. These healing energy generators are: 1. your breathing and 2. gentle and soothing tactile stimulation. The methods described in the exercises below are called "comfort transfers" (Zarren and Eimer 2001).

**6.18A:** Focus on any part of your body that feels comfortable. Notice the nature of the more comfortable sensations in that part of your body. Let yourself become more and more relaxed with each and every normal breath you take. Now, with your breath, spread those comfortable sensations to the part of your body that needs more comfort. Each breath moving more of the comfort toward where it is most needed. Allow the comfort to flow to where you want it. Breathe the comfort from where you found it to where you need it most. There is an unlimited supply of this comfort at its source, where it came from. You can have as much as you need. How is your body feeling now?

> **Self-suggestion.** *I breathe comfort from one part of my body to another.*

**6.18B:** Place one or the other palm down on your leg or thigh. Concentrate and become aware of a strong pulse in one or more fingertips of that hand. When you are aware of the pulse, let the pulsing be a generator for feelings of warmth and make that hand feel warm. When the hand feels warm, place the hand and your strongly pulsing fingertips on the affected part of your body and spread the healing energy of the strong pulse and the warmth into this area where you need more comfort. Concentrate on increasing the warmth in this area. At what point do you become aware that the affected area is much more comfortable?

> **Self-suggestion.** *I keep my hand on the pulse of growing comfort.*

**6.18C:** Raise one of your forearms at a forty-five degree angle, bent at the elbow with your elbow resting on the arm of a chair or on a flat surface. Stare at your hand suspended in the air and recall how numb that hand would feel if you immersed it in a bucket of ice water or if you submersed it in wet, freezing snow for about five minutes. At the moment when you are aware of that numb feeling in your hand, place the hand lightly on the affected area of your body. Spread the icy cold numbness into the affected area so that it penetrates deeply. You will know when the numbness has penetrated deeply enough because the area will feel more comfortable. How did that work? What was that like?

> **Self-suggestion.** *I can create icy cold numbness to neutralize the pain.*

**6.18D:** This exercise is a variation of the above exercise. Place one of your hands palm down on the area of your body that hurts. If you can't reach, rest your hand on a part of your body you can easily reach and do the rest of this exercise in your imagination. It will work just as well either way. Feel the temperature of the affected area. Is it warm or cold? Notice if the area feels like it is pulsating or throbbing. Does the area feel hard or soft to the touch? Now, if the area feels warm or burning, spread the warm or burning feelings into your hand. As you spread this heat out of the affected area and into your hand, this leaves a feeling of cool numbness in the affected area. Shake the heat out of your hand and dissipate it into the air. Now concentrate on the increasing feeling of icy cool numbness in the affected area and the increased comfort there.

If the affected area feels cold, spread the warmth from your hand into the affected area. Begin by concentrating on the pulsing in one or more of your fingertips. Let this pulsing become a generator for a growing feeling of warmth in your hand. When your hand feels noticeably warmer, spread that warmth into the affected area and feel that area becoming warmer and more and more comfortable. How did that work? What was that like?

> **Self-suggestion.** *I use my hand to create comfort where there was discomfort.*

**6.18E:** Place the palm of one of your hands on an area of your body closest to some internal physical problem that you know is maintaining your pain. Now, apply light pressure to the skin surface. This light pressure will penetrate deeply in your body into the area that needs healing the most. It will direct your immune system to concentrate healing energy to that needy place. This method can be effective in reducing pain that is internal and related to physical trauma or disease.

> **Self-suggestion.** *I can concentrate healing energy into the area that needs it most.*

Please note, as I mentioned above, that with any of these exercises, if you cannot reach the affected area, that needn't be a problem. Just place your hand on a part of your body that is closest to the affected area or easiest for you to reach. Intend that the healing energy and comfort transfers reach the affected areas and they will.

## Exercise 6.19: Opposing Qualities Technique

Go back and look at the pain descriptors you picked as being most characteristic of your pain on the Pain Description Questionnaire in chapter 2. Then look at the opposing qualities that you marked as having the most meaning to you. In this exercise, you're going to use your imagination to transform these pain sensations into those opposing sensations associated with comfort. Those opposing qualities can serve as comfort cues.

**6.19A:** Start with the easiest pain sensations to transform. These would be pain sensations that are significant, but not the most intense; perhaps no more than a 7 on your 0 to 10 scale. Recall that you only searched for opposing qualities for pain descriptors that you rated as 5 or higher. These would also be pain sensations that have compelling opposing qualities. So begin by focusing on a single pain characteristic. Imagine that characteristic diminishing and being replaced by its most compelling opposing quality. Do this for several other pain sensations. What does doing this feel like for you? What kind of difference does it make?

> **Self-suggestion.** *I imagine the main pain sensations diminishing and being replaced by their opposing qualities.*

**6.19B:** Now focus on the pain sensations in an area of your body that hurts. Study the sensations. Notice if you can experience the different aspects of these sensations. Are there words to describe them? Or just images, pictures, or feelings? How about sounds, tastes, or smells? Pain is a form of energy. Energy can be converted or transformed from one form into another.

Is it possible for you to imagine the color of your pain being diluted? Its strength being subdued? The space it takes up shrinking? Its depth diminishing? Your soreness subsiding? Your aching turning into a more gentle pressure, and the pressure gradually lessening? Your stinging turning into an itch? Your itching getting soothed? Feelings of heaviness being diminished by a lifting off of some sort of weight or pressure? Stabbing sensations being diminished as you gain control over your image of whatever you visualize as causing those stabbing sensations?

Fatigue being replaced by energy as you recall what it feels like to feel alert, refreshed, interested, energized, and comfortable? Stiffness and tightness loosening and unwinding? The surging or shooting of pain slowing down and changing into a trickling or gentle and smooth flowing? Any cutting or tearing being mended? Gnawing changing into a soothing rubbing or massaging? Pounding quieting? Soreness healing? Jumpiness calming? Heat being cooled and comforted?

Annoyance turning into neutrality? Punishment being replaced by forgiveness? Cruelty being replaced by kindness and compassion? Fear being replaced by courage? Strain being replaced by feelings of resourcefulness? Depression being replaced by encouragement and hope? Hurt being replaced by comfort? Stubbornness being replaced by flexibility?

So, what do you notice? What was that like? Write your responses in your notebook.

> **Self-suggestion.** *All of the pain's sensory qualities are being neutralized or being transformed into and replaced by their opposites.*

## Exercise 6.20: Taking the Pain Apart

First of all, focus all of your attention on the pain sensations in an area of your body. What do the sensations feel like? Let your inner mind bring up images that represent these feelings. Wait for an image to come up. Does this image have a shape? A color? A tint? How bright versus dull is it? Is it light or dark? Does the image have a texture? Is it smooth or rough? Hard or soft? How much of an area does the pain cover? Does the area have firm boundaries, or are they fuzzy or blurred, or are there no boundaries at all? Is it stationary or is it spreading? Is there depth to it? Does it penetrate below the surface of your skin? How deep? Are the sensations and images changing, or are they pretty motionless and fixed?

What do the sensations remind you of? Where do you feel they are coming from? Let your inner mind bring up to a conscious level an image or idea about the cause or origin of the sensations. In other words, what is generating them? Wait for an answer. It may come up in the form of another thought, word, sound, image, picture, or feeling. What comes up for you?

Now focus your attention on the qualities of the pain sensations that you identified; for example, their shape or size. Can you change the shape or size in some way? Can you shrink the area the sensations cover? Can you make the texture smoother? Can you move the pain to another part of your body where it's less uncomfortable, such as perhaps your small toe?

What about the color of the pain? What is your favorite color associated with healing and comfort? Can you get the pain color to change into this more comfortable, pleasant color? Perhaps you can make the color of the pain fade. Now, if the sensations remind you of something real, like electricity or a knife or a jackhammer or a drill, can you take charge of this? Can you imagine removing the knife, turning off the electricity, or getting the hammering or drilling to stop?

Think about what makes you feel more comfortable; what diminishes the pain, what gives you relief. Is it applying ice packs? Moist heat? A warm shower? A hot bath? A relaxing whirlpool? Having a massage? Lying in the sun on the beach, in the park, by the pool, or in your back yard? Taking a good nap? Stretching? Exercising in your favorite way? For example, walking briskly, swimming, bicycling, lifting weights? Taking medicine? Can you imagine these relief factors going to the roots of the symptoms? To their cause? Can you imagine them soothing the roots of the problem? Can you imagine and feel your medicine working?

Now, how was that experience? What kind of difference did this exercise make?

> **Self-suggestion.** *I direct my mind to visualize what diminishes the discomfort and brings relief.*

## Exercise 6.21: Changing Your Perception of Discomfort Intensity

Begin by rating your current level of discomfort on a 0 to 10 scale. A rating of 0 represents the "most comfortable" and 10 the "least comfortable." Take yourself into relaxation and self-hypnosis using whichever method you choose. When you know you're in hypnosis, concentrate on taking yourself even deeper into relaxation. When you're satisfied with how deeply relaxed you have become, concentrate on taking yourself down to a number that represents a lower level of discomfort. Take as much time as you need. When you reach that number you will know it, as you'll feel more comfortable.

Now that you know how to do it, take yourself down another few numbers on the scale. You will know when you are there. Then linger there for a while and enjoy that new, greater level of comfort. When you're ready, you can even move down a few more numbers to an even greater level of comfort. You can get as comfortable as your inner mind is ready for you to get, and that's great. How was that? What was that experience like?

Whatever your experience with this exercise, it helps you to build a memory of a new level of comfort that you will be able to reach again and again and eventually maintain. Each time you do this exercise, you will be able to get more comfortable for longer and longer periods of time.

**Self-suggestion.** *I can borrow back the memory of greater comfort whenever I need to.*

## Exercise 6.22: Healing Imagery Steps

Begin by visualizing the physical cause of your discomfort, what is going on in your body that is generating the signals of pain up your spinal cord to your brain. When you get the image, let the index finger of your nondominant hand lift up as a signal to yourself that you've locked in on this image. Then relax your index finger.

Now visualize your medical treatment, or the medicine you're taking for pain relief, working. Notice what comes in to your conscious mind. Perhaps, in your mind's eye, you can see your medication being carried through your bloodstream to the parts of your body that are asking for relief. See, feel, and experience your medication soothing the inflammation, or dissolving the molecules that are responsible for the pain or swelling and lubricating your joints. Experience your medicine sending quiet messages through your nervous system to the central control center in your brain that processes all pain. Feel your medicine replenishing the supply of essential neurochemicals that your body needs more of. Observe and sense your body sending appropriate messages to the central control center in your brain to switch off the pain or switch on the appropriate healing mechanism.

Now visualize the application of any remedies that give you relief. For example, the application of ice, moist heat, massage, electrical counterstimulation, and so on.

Now visualize the healing forces of your body and mind; your basic, healing life energy. Get in touch now with this powerful healing life force within you. It's the energy that enables your immune system to fight off infection and protect you from other diseases. It's the energy that maintains the rhythm of your heartbeat, your breathing, all of your vital functions. Where is this energy coming from? What is its source? Is it coming from your breath? Your heart? Your belly? Your back? The base of your spine? Your brain? A higher power? Wait and notice what comes to mind.

Now direct this energetic life force to power up your healing, to energize your medical treatments, to boost every good thing that brings you relief and comfort. You may help this along with your breathing. With each breath you take and each additional word that you read, you let more and more of this healing energy strengthen your treatment and help you to get well. Ask your unconscious to make this happen for you, and let it happen.

Now place your hands palms down, if you can reach, over the area that hurts. If you cannot reach, put your hands anywhere else on your body where you can rest your hands comfortably; for example, your belly, your chest, your legs, your thighs, or your head. Now surround yourself with white light or a light of your favorite color that you associate with healing. There is an unlimited supply. Ask your inner mind to let your body become a transmitter of this healing light energy. Let this light bathe you in its warm, glowing, healing energy. Absorb it into your body from the top of your head, your shoulders, and your back. Let it travel through you. Breathe it through you. Circulate it throughout your body with your breath. Let it concentrate in your hands and from your hands, let it flow out your fingertips and out your palms to where it is most needed in your body. Experience this life-force energy combining with the energy of your treatment and the energy of all those things that give you comfort and relief to heal the cause of your symptoms and pain and to transform your pain into greater comfort. When you know that you have done enough healing work for now, that you're feeling more comfortable, and the qualities of the pain have changed just enough so that you can notice a positive difference, let your nondominant index finger lift up slowly to verify that this is so. Then relax the finger.

When your deepest mind is satisfied that it has sent enough healing energy for now to where it is most needed in your body, and is fully aware of how much comfort you have now, and satisfied that it can maintain your new comfort level for some time after this exercise, your eyes blink several times and then open wide and return to focus . You come back feeling fully alert, sound in mind, sound in body, and in full control of your feelings.

**Self-suggestion.** *I send healing energy to the areas in my body where it is most needed.*

## Some Additional Distortion Self-Suggestions

The list below provides you with choices of distortion self-suggestions to help you transform or alter your pain symptoms. As I instructed you to do earlier with the decatastrophizing, deep relaxation, and direction self-suggestions, simply choose two or three of the suggestions in the list below to read to yourself several times before you enter self-hypnosis from now on. If you choose at this point to work with distortion, focus on these active sensory imagination self-suggestions and put aside the previous self-suggestions that you may have been working with up until now. The guiding principle bears repeating:

Work with a few self-suggestions repeatedly for a while, and then switch to several others. By working in this way, you will find it easy to remain focused, and you will succeed in imprinting the suggestions you choose in your unconscious.

1.  I am interrupting the transmission of pain sensations from my [body part] to my brain.

2.  I am turning down the intensity of my discomfort.

3.  I am turning the discomfort switch to the off position on my electrical control panel in my brain's central control room.

4.  I am changing the channel on the pain.

5.  The area that had been hurting is now cool and comfortable.

6.  The area that had been hurting is now warm and flexible.

7.  I am spreading comfort from one part of my body to another.

8.  I am filtering the hurt out of the pain.

9.  The pain sensations are changing. They are getting weaker.

10. I can loosen the vise of the pain.

11. I can turn down the flame of the pain.

12. I can turn down the pain dial to a lower setting.

# ◎ Dissociation: The Sixth D

Finally, we reach dissociation, the sixth D. *Dissociation* is the "pure gold" of all self-hypnosis strategies for getting out of pain. Basically, the coping strategy of dissociation means detaching, disconnecting, and disengaging yourself from pain. It means isolating or separating the pain from you and you from the pain.

Dissociation depends on the idea that the mind is made up of two parts (Zarren and Eimer 2001). One part we call the conscious mind. You have control over your conscious mind, and it controls conscious behavior; things you can't do without knowing that you are doing them. Behavior and experience can't change without the cooperation of the conscious mind. So, it is important for your conscious mind to be fully aware of all of the important issues relating to coping effectively with chronic pain. The other part of the mind we call the unconscious, the subconscious, or the inner mind. All three names mean the same thing. The unconscious controls all of your automatic functions. These include your breathing, heartbeat, pulse rate, blood flow, digestion; all of the things that keep you alive that you pay little or no attention to. They are automatic.

The unconscious also controls all the things that you do every day automatically without thinking much about them (Zarren and Eimer 2001). These things include your habits and automatic behaviors; for example, which side of the bed you sleep on, which shoe you put on first when you get dressed in the morning, driving (if you drive), daily maintenance chores, such as taking out the trash, putting dirty dishes in the dishwasher, running your washer and dryer, and so forth. Your unconscious or inner mind also controls your coping habits; for example, how you talk to yourself, how you handle anger and frustration, how you cope with your pain, and so forth.

Dissociating pain, that is, isolating or separating the pain from you and you from the pain, creates a very special situation that is one of the main characteristics of hypnosis. This involves freeing your conscious mind from the immediate perception of pain and relegating or transferring the pain to your unconscious. Your unconscious is entrusted with the job of holding your pain while your conscious mind enjoys freedom from pain. Part of you gets comfortable and pain-free, while another part of you, your inner mind, remains aware of the pain on an unconscious level.

As with the strategy of distortion, the intentional employment of the strategy of dissociation requires that you believe in your creative imagination and active sensory imagination. To understand dissociation fully, however, we need to examine several examples of normal, everyday dissociation.

### Everyday, Spontaneous Dissociation

We all have the ability to dissociate to greater or lesser degrees. One rather undramatic example of everyday spontaneous dissociation is when you are driving your car to and from a familiar location. If you have taken the same route countless times before, you don't have to think about which turns to make, what streets to take, etc. You can use the driving time to listen to the radio or review your day. You mentally dissociate from the task at hand, driving. While your unconscious carries out the rote, overlearned task of operating your vehicle and ensuring you arrive at your destination safely, your conscious mind is free to go somewhere else. Only if something unexpected happens that draws your conscious attention do you turn it back to the driving task.

When you learn something new it typically requires all of your conscious attention. Remember when you first learned to read? Now you no longer have to think about such things. It's automatic and unconscious.

In fact, you can read and write and think about something else at the same time.

How can you make pain mostly unconscious? The answer is by learning and practicing the basic self-hypnosis coping skills we have already covered so that they become automatic habits. By practicing these skills over and over again, their use will become spontaneous and automatic.

## Spontaneous Dissociation as a Survival Mechanism

Many people who have survived a life-threatening motor vehicle accident have reported that while the accident was happening, time seemed to slow down; that it seemed as if everything was occurring in slow motion. In my own motor vehicle accident, that was my experience also. Somehow or other while the accident was happening, I disconnected from any fear and my body's rush of adrenaline. This allowed me to stay in control of my vehicle. After the accident, I experienced an intense rush of fear that disoriented me, and in a different way I dissociated again. I found myself standing out in the cold (it was December) by my totalled vehicle, shaking—but it felt like I was not in my body. I felt disconnected from myself. I continued to feel detached throughout the trip to the emergency room and my stay there.

The point I want to make is that spontaneous, unplanned dissociation is a survival mechanism that, in a dangerous situation, allows you to stay in control by being in two places at once. You split or divide your consciousness. In my car accident, part of me was maintaining control of my careening vehicle, while another part of me was observing everything happening in slow motion. Similarly, when you are able to harness the power of dissociation to control your chronic pain, part of you can remain comfortable so that you can do what you want to do (such as relaxing, doing self-hypnosis, performing some other activity), while another part of you (your unconscious mind) holds the pain sensations. The desired result of dividing your consciousness for this purpose is that you remain conscious of what you want to be conscious of (comfort) and unconscious of the discomfort.

## Using Dissociation as a Coping Tool

So now that you know something about dissociation, how can you actually employ it to cope with pain? The exercises below provide a number of methods.

Once again, follow the same instructions that I gave you before for using the exercises in distraction and distortion, and experience how pleasant and easy controlled dissociation can be.

## Exercise 6.23: Pure Dissociation Exercise

**6.23A:** When you are fully present in the front of your mind, you are unaware of the sensations in the back of your mind. So, while you remain fully present in the front of your mind, you can temporarily relegate the pain to the back of your mind. When you know that all of the pain has been placed in the back of your mind, your nondominant index finger will slowly lift up to signal this. Then relax the finger. At that point, you may hear vague, faraway noises associated with your pain, or you may feel very slight sensations that are just vague echoes of the pain sensations in the back of your mind. How does that feel? What is that like?

> *Dear Inner Mind: Would you be willing to hold the pain temporarily so that my conscious mind can be aware of what it feels like to be comfortable? Thank you, my Inner Mind, for cooperating.*

**6.23B:** Put your pain in a closet and lock the door. There are many closets in your subconscious or inner mind. These are places where experiences and memories are stored. They are not real closets, but they have some qualities in common with real closets. They have only so much space to store memories. If you exceed their capacity, you need to locate new closet space. Similar things are kept in the same closet, unless you are very unorganized. When you put things in a closet, you are able to clear space outside the closet and make room for other things. So, when you lock your pain experience up in one of the closets within your inner mind, you make available space in your outer, conscious mind for comfort. The rooms in your house feel more comfortable when they are free of clutter, when junk is put away in your closets. Similarly, you feel more comfortable, when your conscious mind, the front of your mind, is free of pain; when the pain is locked away in the closets in the back of your mind.

Now as you know, there comes a time when you need to devote some energy to cleaning out your closets. Similarly, you need to devote some time and energy to doing your self-hypnosis to clean out your mental closets of pain, tension, stress, and discomfort. You feel so much lighter and freer and so much more relieved afterwards.

> *Dear Inner Mind: Would you be willing to make some inner space to hold the pain temporarily so that space is freed up in my outer conscious mind to enjoy some comfort? Thank you, my Inner Mind, for cooperating.*

## Exercise 6.24: An Out of Body Exercise

Can you imagine floating off to a very nice place while you leave your painful body parts behind for a while? For example, can you imagine your consciousness floating out of your physical body and hovering above your body so that you see your body from above? This is like taking a sort of brief spirit trip and then returning to your body. When you do this, you leave your pain behind for a while. When you merge back into your body, you will find that the pain is worn out and weaker. Let your inner mind review this as a possibility, and do it if it feels right. What was that like?

Can you temporarily forget about the pain and float off to a beach somewhere? (Only if you like the beach!) If you don't like the beach, can you float off to another place you do find pleasant? Let your inner mind review this as a possibility, and do it if it feels right. What was that like?

**Self-suggestion.** *When I permit my conscious mind to float away to a pleasant place, I forget about the pain.*

## Exercise 6.25: A Pain Number Blackboard

Visualize a blackboard, and on the blackboard see a number being written. That number reflects the current level of your discomfort. When you see the number, your nondominant index finger will lift. Then relax the finger. That number on this imaginary blackboard influences your comfort level. This is because when the number changes, the pain also changes, and when the pain changes, the number changes. Now direct your inner mind to re-write the number appearing on that blackboard.

Sort of experiment with the numbers, and experience how each number makes you feel. Experiment first with increasing the number and making the pain worse! When you've erased the old number and re-written a higher number, or seen a higher number just appear, let your nondominant index finger lift up slowly all by itself to verify this. Then relax the finger. Make a note to yourself. Because your inner mind can make the numbers go up, your inner mind can also make the numbers go down. So go ahead and see how low your inner mind can make the numbers go, and feel the pain going down with the numbers.

**Self-suggestion.** *I can erase the pain rating I see written on my inner blackboard, and write a lower number. This helps me become more comfortable.*

# Exercise 6.26: Dialogue with the Pain

Focus directly on the pain. Concentrate on the sensations and just notice what happens, what you are experiencing. Notice if the sensations change in some noticeable way. After you've concentrated for a little while on those sensations, describe to yourself what is happening and what you're experiencing.

Now invite an image to come to mind that can tell you something useful about the pain, and when such an image comes to mind, please describe it to yourself. Thank your inner mind for bringing that information to your conscious attention.

Now remain deeply relaxed, and concentrate on that image. Ask the image what it is doing and why it's doing it. Talk to that image and search deep down inside yourself to find out what that image means for you and what its purpose is, so that you can learn something useful from it. Imagine that it can answer you in a way that you understand, and when an idea comes up that you feel is important or significant, go over it so that you will remember it. You may write this information down in your notebook now or later.

Now really get in touch with the image and the pain. Talk to it. Say whatever you feel needs to be said. Ask the pain whatever you want to ask it. Make sure the pain hears you and you hear it. Then, wait and see what else comes to mind: thoughts, images, sensations, feelings. Ask the pain what it wants from you. Why it came to be. Where it comes from. What brings it out. What its purpose is. What it needs from you. Wait for it to respond in some way, to answer you. Make a note of the information you have learned.

You may even wish to really get inside the pain and temporarily get into the feeling of being that pain instead of being you. Sort of merge with it, so that you can really experience its point of view. At this point in this exercise, you are the pain, and you can talk back to yourself as the pain, temporarily taking on the pain's voice. And as you do this, just answer with whatever it is that naturally comes from that position. Shift back and forth between the two positions, between being you and being the pain; going back to being yourself and seeing if there is anything else to say to the pain or ask it, and then going back to being the pain. Continue with this dialogue as long as there remains something useful for you to learn right now.

Lastly, express your appreciation and thanks to the inner part of you that has willingly shared this information with you. Ask the inner pain image if it would be willing to work with you from now on, for both of your benefits, to better understand and reduce your discomfort and your suffering, and to help you get well and function better. Listen to, see, and feel what comes up. Be aware of the responses you get and how you feel. Record your responses and experience in your notebook.

**Self-suggestion.** *I can carry on an inner dialogue with my pain and even become friends with it.*

# Exercise 6.27: Awareness, Analysis, and Alteration

Begin by focusing directly on your pain. Concentrate on the sensations, and just notice what the pain feels like. Notice it's qualities, attributes, or features. What color is it? Is it hot or cool or cold? What shape is it? How large an area does it take up? Is it just on the surface or does it penetrate deeply? Is its texture smooth or rough? Is it hard or soft? Stationary or moving? Light or heavy? Is it pressing? Is it uniform and in one piece, or made up of many parts or pieces? What does it feel like it's made up of? Just note these things.

Now stay with the pure sensations for a while, and think about how they feel. And as you pay attention to how they feel, just notice, just watch, just observe how they begin to change, and observe the changes. The sensory qualities of the pain will change, because no pain ever stays exactly the same, and no pain lasts forever. So just notice what the sensations are, and notice how they change.

Stay focused inside and notice the changes as they happen, and also notice whether there is anything that you can bring in that might change it even more in the direction of greater comfort. What might you bring in to change the feeling into one of greater comfort?

You may want to imagine the color of the pain growing lighter or the area of the pain growing smaller. Lighter and lighter in color, smaller and smaller in size. And when the pain has become very light and very small, perhaps it disappears and is eliminated through one of the passageways of the body. It may float out of your ears, or out of your fingertips, or maybe it falls like rain out the bottoms of your feet.

Take all the time you need to concentrate on what's happening so that you can learn something useful that is associated with increased comfort.

Now, if you could give yourself something that would totally block the pain, totally relieve the discomfort, totally oppose the sensations and qualities you have noted, sort of like a pain antidote, what would it feel like? Take all the time you need to go deep inside and let your inner mind bring up an image or symbol that carries relief and comfort. When your inner mind has come up with such an image, let your nondominant index finger lift up all by itself as a signal that a symbol has come to mind. Then relax the finger.

Now breathe right through that pain and right through that healing image, and as you breathe deeply, breathe that pain antidote image right through the pain. Feel your breath moving through those sensations and feelings of pain. Notice how the sensations change, as you mix the pain antidote with the pain, as you breathe through all of this, really working it with your breathing.

You know what brings relief. As you continue to breathe deeply and easily, remaining deeply relaxed, notice if the sensations cool down or warm up, change color, or perhaps change in temperature from a hot red to a cool blue, or from an icy cold white to a warm pink. Perhaps you notice the area that contained the pain shrinking in size, changing in texture from rough to smooth, changing shape, moving up to the surface, becoming less intense or less concentrated, becoming softer, lighter, and less pressing, breaking apart, or becoming smoother.

The main idea is that there is no limit to what you can, with your inner mind and your imagination, do to a physical sensation. Pain is just a sensation, and sensations keep changing. No sensations ever remain exactly the same. So you can explore and change the sensations. You can explore what changes work for you, describing them to yourself when you're ready and writing them down in your notebook.

> **Self-suggestion.** *As I become more aware of my pain's qualities, I gain greater control over them. I can analyze these qualities without judging them and alter them in the direction of greater comfort.*

## Exercise 6.28: Direct Suggestions for Pain Alleviation

Turn your attention to your pain sensations, and go deep into relaxation and hypnosis by counting slowly down from ten to one. With each number that you count, you'll find yourself going deeper, and as you go deeper, as you count slowly down to one, the pain will begin to diminish, and it will become less and less as you say each number. The pain will fade as the numbers go down, and when you say the number one, the pain will have almost faded totally away. When you reach the count of one, all unnecessary pain will be totally gone. You'll be left with only that amount of pain that your inner mind feels it needs to perform the protective signal function that pain is meant to perform, and no more pain than that.

So, just count down slowly to yourself, listening to the numbers. Let yourself go, and enjoy the experience of feeling much more comfortable as you go much deeper into relaxation and hypnosis and as the pain diminishes and fades away. As you go deeper with each number, you feel better. 10 … 9 … 8 … 7 … 6 … 5 … 4 … 3 … 2 … 1. You're much, much more deeply relaxed.

When your conscious mind becomes aware of the increased level of comfort you feel, when all unnecessary pain is totally gone, your nondominant index finger will slowly rise all by itself as a signal to let you know that it feels "yes." Then relax the finger.

> **Self-suggestion.** *When I count from 10 down 1, I count down to much greater comfort.*

## Exercise 6.29: Hypnotic Dreaming

Imagine that you are standing at the top of a stairway. There are twenty steps to the bottom. At the bottom of the stairs, there's a room that you can enter, and in this room there's a very comfortable couch. When you enter this room, you can lie down on that couch and have a hypnotic dream. So, walk down this stairway, counting down slowly as you do, one number for each stair. And when you get to the bottom, open the door to the room, enter the room, and lie down on the couch.

Whether you choose to keep your eyes open or closed, you feel very drowsy when you lie down on this couch. It's very easy to let yourself drift into a sleep-like pattern, moving into a hypnotic dream. It will be a dream like the kind you have at night, and it will somehow deal with your pain problem. Your dream will suggest a solution to your pain problem. As soon as you begin dreaming, your nondominant index finger will slowly rise all by itself and then relax. And as soon as the dream comes to an end, your thumb on the same hand will slowly rise all by itself and then relax. And when you complete the dream, you'll awaken feeling alert and refreshed, and you'll remember the dream in detail and be able to describe it in your notebook. So, pleasant dreams.

**Self-suggestion.** *I can have an unconscious dream that will suggest a solution to some aspect of my pain problem.*

## Exercise 6.30: The Zarren Shadow Method

The following method was developed by Jordan Zarren (Zarren and Eimer 2001). It is based on the idea of detaching from physical feelings in the body. It invokes the idea of a *shadow*.

A shadow is attached to your body, to your arms, your feet, or wherever you choose. It is a part of you, but it's not inside of you. Imagine your shadow. Then imagine yourself merging with your shadow. This allows you to feel dissociated or outside of your physical body, although you are still connected. Doing this is a way of inducing an altered state of consciousness or trance. It allows you to sense yourself floating slightly out of your body. This way of dissociating or detaching from your body and the pain is a way to help you feel better, to feel more comfortable.

You can experience further dissociation, detachment from the discomfort, and greater comfort by putting pain into your shadow; that is, out of your "real body" and into your "shadow body." You can further detach that shadow from your total being even though it's still a part of you. You will enjoy this hypnotic experience. Practice it as part of your self-hypnosis. It will increase your control.

The level of comfort you attain will continue for some time after this altered state experience. Practicing this technique as part of your own self-hypnosis will improve your skill in detaching and disconnecting from the pain.

**Self-suggestion.** *I can imagine my body's shadow and displace some of the pain into my shadow.*

## Exercise 6.31: The Movie-Theater Technique

This method is adapted from Brown and Fromm (1986).

First relax yourself and get comfortable. When you are feeling more relaxed and comfortable, imagine that you are sitting in a movie theater. The screen is blank, and you are curious about what will soon appear on the screen. In a few moments the movie will begin. The movie will be a short scene about one kind of situation that you have to deal with a lot in your daily life because of your persistent pain. The scene will show somebody like you who knows exactly how to cope with that situation so that the pain does not disrupt that person's life. You are curious to see what works for that person. By watching the scene you will learn something useful. Now you are waiting for the scene to start. When it starts, the index finger of your nondominant hand will lift up slowly all by itself and then relax. Watch the scene through to the end. When the scene ends, your thumb on that hand will lift up and then relax. In the future, whenever you find yourself in a similar situation, thoughts about the coping strategy you have seen will automatically come into your mind. What came up for you?

**Self-suggestion.** *I can watch a movie in the theater of my mind that provides a solution to some aspect of my pain problem.*

## Exercise 6.32: The Split-Screen Technique

This method is adapted from Spiegel and Spiegel (1978).

Imagine a screen in front of you divided into three parts, left, right, and middle. The middle screen is the "receiving screen." That's where thoughts or memories are projected initially. If they are neutral they remain there. If they are negative or bad, then they are transferred to the left screen. If they are positive or good, then they are transferred to the right screen. The middle is also the storage area for trivia or irrelevant thoughts that come along. The right and left screens are for charged or polarized thoughts, the good and the bad, the right and the wrong.

This screen becomes a means for you to neutralize emotionally charged problems resulting from your pain, by first receiving the information and then separating out the positive and negative aspects of the situation. This assists you in problem solving. First, you need to just gather information about your problem without making any judgments. So, the information is received in the middle, neutral screen. Then you need to sort through the information. You find what's useful, what's helpful, and put it in the right screen for later reference. You take out what's unhelpful or negative, and place it in the left screen. It remains contained there where it can do less harm.

This method also allows you to gain a clearer, more balanced perspective on your problem. It enables you to see that it's not all bad. In fact, the more that you focus on the neutral in the middle and the positive that's on the right, the less impact the negative that's left has. Somehow, by focusing on the neutral in the middle and the positive that's right, you experience the negative diminishing. The triple screen also helps you gain greater insight and control over the situation and your symptoms.

By examining the different aspects of the situation up on the screen, you may find that what you thought was negative really is positive and is right for you. You may also find that what you thought was positive belongs on the left part of the screen. And whatever you continue to be unsure of can stay neutral, in the middle.

**Self-suggestion.** *I use the three-paneled split screen in the theater of my mind to neutralize discomfort, and then I sort out the positive and negative aspects of the situation.*

## Exercise 6.33: The Crystal Ball Technique

You don't need a crystal ball for this exercise, but if you happen to have one it will work great as a focusing object. If not, you can easily imagine that you are staring at a crystal ball about eight inches in diameter sitting on a table or shelf not too far in front of you. Alternatively, you can get a clear glass or crystal bowl and fill it with water, placing it on a table or shelf not too far away.

Focus your visual attention on this object. As you stare at this concentration object, visualize as manifesting within the crystal ball or water bowl an experience that you associate with comfort and healing. Choose an experience that is associated with getting better, getting well. When your inner mind accesses the right experience, your eyes will close, and you will enter self-hypnosis and have a dream about that healing experience. When you are through dreaming, and when your deepest mind knows that it can maintain the comfort associated with the dream and continue to process what you have learned in this exercise, blink your eyes, open them wide, and come back fully alert, sound in mind, sound in body, and in control of your feelings.

What was that like? What did you learn? Write your insights in your notebook.

> **Self-suggestion.** *I gaze into my inner mind and come up with experiences that help me to heal and get well.*

## Exercise 6.34: Body Lights Imagery

Ernest Rossi and David Cheek (Rossi and Cheek 1988) developed a dissociative hypnotic imagery technique for relieving painful symptoms. The following is a step-by-step adaptation of their approach:

1. Imagine standing in front of a full-length mirror and seeing tiny colored lights in different parts of your body. These colors represent physical sensations, including pain. Your index finger on your nondominant hand will lift up when you can see the total picture and then your finger will relax.

2. Scan your entire body and note what each colored light stands for or represents.

3. Select the least painful body part to begin doing some therapeutic work. Let your inner mind go back to a time when that body light stood for comfort (or any opposing quality to the pain). When you are there, your index finger will lift up and then relax.

4. Now shift forward in time to the first moment when the light that now stands for pain took the place of the light that stood for comfort. Your index finger will lift when you arrive at that moment and then relax. When you are there, please note your age and what is going on in your life.

5. Is there any good reason now why you have to continue having pain in that body part? If the answer that comes up is "yes," it is important to explore the reasons.

6. If the answer that comes up is "no," ask your inner mind the following question: Now that you are aware of what is happening, is your inner mind willing to let you turn off or turn down that light, and with it that pain, and continue the healing process? If the answer is "no," what stands in the way?

7. If your inner mind is not willing to allow the pain to be turned off or down, you will need to explore the factors that stand in the way of pain relief. We will cover several ways to do that in chapter 8.

8. If your inner mind is willing to allow the pain to be turned off or down, go ahead now and imagine a future time when you are no longer suffering from pain in that body part. When you are there, your index finger will lift and then relax, and you will see the month, day, and year as though written on a chalkboard right in front of you.

9. I suggest that you practice orienting to this future time and rehearse imagining the associated sensations of comfort.

10. Repeat the above steps for other, more painful body parts so that you can gradually work your way up a sort of hierarchy of increasingly painful body parts and feel more and more comfortable in more and more parts of your body.

**Self-suggestion.** *I imagine the colored lights that are associated with discomfort in the parts of my body that hurt. I also imagine replacing those lights with lights of a different color that are associated with greater comfort and healing.*

# Exercise 6.35: LeCron's "Control Panel of Light Switches"

One great technique described by Leslie LeCron (1964) involves visualizing a control panel of light switches with a different colored light bulb above each switch. Each switch goes to a different part of your body. This set of suggestions puts you back in charge.

Visualize the area of your body that you want to work with. Now imagine a control panel of light switches with a different colored light bulb above each switch. The index finger on your nondominant hand will lift up when you get this image and then will relax.

Next, locate the switch that is connected to the area of your body that you have chosen to work with now. This switch controls the sensations in that body part. That switch sends nerve impulses from your brain down to that part of you and from that part back up to your brain. When you lock in this image, your nondominant index finger will lift up and then relax. What color is the light above that switch?

Now, turn this one switch off, and see the colored light above the switch go out. It may go out right away, or it may get dimmer and dimmer before it goes out completely. You may also hear the click of the switch as you turn the switch off. You may see the light go out, hear the switch go off, or both. You may or may not immediately have a sensation of numbness or diminished sensation in the area you are working with. What is most important is to experience the diminished discomfort first at an unconscious or inner level. You will know that this is happening, because the index finger of your nondominant hand will lift up and then relax as a signal. By repeating this exercise, you experience greater comfort on a conscious level.

It's important that you take the time to practice this exercise because, by doing so, you are conditioning your inner mind to be less sensitive to pain. The more you practice this exercise, the better you become at using this method to diminish your discomfort. Your success in using this exercise will also depend on your mental attitude. Doubts on your part will only impede your ability to get it to work and to get relief. Skepticism prevents self-suggestion from taking root, while positive belief promotes your ability to accomplish something worthwhile.

> **Self-suggestion.** *I can switch off the sensations of discomfort that flow to my body part that needs greater comfort.*

## Some Additional Dissociation Self-Suggestions

The list below provides you with more choices of dissociation and imaginative fantasy self-suggestions to help you remove yourself or distance yourself from your pain. As I instructed you to do earlier with the decatastrophizing, deep relaxation, direction, and distortion self-suggestions, simply choose two or three of the suggestions in the list below to read to yourself several times before you enter self-hypnosis from now on. If you choose at this point to work with dissociation, focus on these active sensory imagination self-suggestions, and put aside the previous self-suggestions that you may have been working with up until now. The guiding principle bears mentioning again: Work with a few self-suggestions repeatedly for a while, and then switch to several others. By working in this way, you will find it easy to remain focused, and you will succeed in imprinting the suggestions you choose in your unconscious.

1.  I can remember a time when I feel very comfortable.

2.  I can remember when I forgot about pain.

3.  When I'm having a good time and enjoying myself, time flies.

4.  I am a secret agent (or soldier, or police officer) who has been wounded doing a very important assignment. I can get through this and complete my assignment successfully.

5.  I got this pain while saving someone's life.

6.  I got this pain from an injury I sustained during combat.

7.   I can dispassionately observe this pain and objectively describe it like a scientist.

8.   This is not my body in pain!

9.   I can have a pleasant daydream.

10.  I experience a small amount of "pure pain" at a tolerable level.

11.  I have the key to the master pain control panel located in my brain.

12.  I can operate a pain dimmer switch in my brain.

13.  I can turn down the pain intensity rheostat in my brain as much as I need.

14.  I can ignore false alarms and respond to genuine alarms.

15.  I can turn down the volume on my pain.

# SEVEN

## Change Your Pain Experience

*The unconscious part of your mind knows the source of your problem and knows what it needs to solve it . . . and I don't know if your unconscious mind will share with your conscious mind that source or just solve the problem without your conscious mind knowing how it was solved.*

**—Milton H. Erickson, M.D.**

The exercises in the last two chapters have provided you with a notable number of alternative ways to reduce and relieve your pain. The exercises in chapter 5 focused on conscious thinking and behavioral coping strategies. Those exercises do not require much in the way of hypnotic relaxation, absorption, focused attention, and imagination, at least not to the degree that the exercises in chapter 6 do. You can achieve success using the exercises in chapter 5 mainly with the cooperation of your conscious mind.

You'll gain success using the exercises in chapter 6 by consciously developing your self-hypnosis skills and conditioning your unconscious mind. Doing this is simple. Practice your self-hypnosis using the method from chapter 4 that you have chosen. Read through all of the exercises in chapter 6 several times. If you wish, you may also tape record the ones you choose and listen to the tape several times. Whether you read or listen to the exercises, the ideas, images, and suggestions that make sense to you and that are acceptable to you automatically will be reinforced each and every time you read or listen to them. Each hypnotic coping strategy in chapter 6 is followed by a positive, helpful self-suggestion that summarizes the essence of that strategy. They will be further reinforced and strengthened each and every time you do your own self-hypnosis using the method you have chosen. The suggestions in the preceding exercises that make sense to you have already been accepted by your unconscious. Each time that you read them or listen to them on tape they will become further fixed in place or imprinted in your unconscious.

# ◎ How to Use Self-Suggestions Effectively

In chapter 5, I explained how to come up with more functional and stress-reducing ways of thinking about stressful situations. I mentioned that the positive thoughts you come up with can provide you with material for constructing specific suggestions to give yourself in self-hypnosis. Both in chapter 5 and 6, we covered numerous thinking, behavioral, distraction, and imagination coping methods. Your practice of self-hypnosis will reinforce the coping methods that appeal to you. Also, for any of these methods, you can create pertinent self-suggestions to give yourself in your normal waking state or while you are in self-hypnosis. Alternatively, you may choose to use the self-suggestions that are given with each of the hypnotic coping strategies in chapter 6.

It's easy to create your own self-suggestions. You select the idea that you want to impress upon your inner mind. Then, you create a simple, brief, specific, and direct statement that communicates that idea using language that employs your preferred sensory systems. ·

**Review Chapters 5 and 6.** After you read the following material on how to construct self-suggestions, it will be a good idea to go back over the exercises in the preceding two chapters to obtain material to create pertinent, individualized self-suggestions. There is a lot of material in the preceding two chapters because I want to give you ample opportunity to choose the coping methods that feel right. You can adopt or modify the self-suggestions provided with each exercise or create your own. Because you choose them or create them, they will work for you.

## *Your Unconscious Is Already Working*

The exercises in the previous three chapters, actually the information in all of the chapters up to this point, have planted seeds in your unconscious that are already growing and cultivating the basis for continuing pain relief and greater comfort. Each and every time you read, reread, and reexperience the preceding exercises, the experience waters and nourishes the positive coping ideas implanted in your unconscious and reinforces the strength of those suggested ideas.

# ◎ Repetition Imprints in Your Unconscious

For each coping strategy exercise that appeals to you, it will be beneficial for you to follow these steps:

1.  Read through and do the exercise. Immediately following that, enter self-hypnosis and remain in self-hypnosis for at least five minutes.

2.  Repeat this process at least three times.

3.  Then, simply read the self-suggestion for that exercise and enter self-hypnosis. Repeat this process twice.

By that point, just reading the self-suggestion will activate the strategy in both your conscious and unconscious minds. The suggestion then can be strengthened and imprinted by entering self-hypnosis or used as a waking-state suggestion.

**Your Unconscious Will Remember.** The famous psychiatrist and clinical hypnosis pioneer, Milton Erickson, M.D., was correct in pointing out that the unconscious knows about things that your conscious mind isn't aware of (Havens 1985). Your conscious and unconscious are separate but interacting systems that operate at different levels of perception and response. Your unconscious operates at multiple levels.

Therefore, you need not worry about remembering everything we have covered because your unconscious mind will remember what's important and use the information when it is needed. Your inner mind is fully aware of how much comfort you have at all times and how much comfort it needs to help you create. Your inner mind is continuing to process what you have read and learned up to this point and will persist in processing what is important to help you continue to find greater comfort.

The material you have read in the preceding chapters and your experience reading through and doing the preceding exercises constitute learning that will be applied to the forces that govern your body. As a result of what you have processed in the preceding exercises, there has been a buildup in your mind and body of certain psychological, physiological, and neurological knowledge and associations that will enable you to gain greater control over your pain. The really important knowledge you have acquired thus far is partly unconscious. It is knowledge that you will be able to use when the appropriate time comes.

# ◎ How to Construct Effective Self-Suggestions

In order to create effective, personal self-suggestions based on your experience and then transform those self-suggestions into your own individual reality, you have to follow certain principles or rules. These rules pertain to the phrasing of the self-suggestions and when to employ them. In this chapter, I am going to teach you how to phrase self-suggestions effectively. Then, I'll explain when to use them. You will learn how to use self-suggestions in the waking state and with self-hypnosis to change your pain experience.

**Rule 1: Use Your Preferred Sensory Systems.** The first rule is to use the language of your preferred sensory systems. That is the language your unconscious understands best and will respond to the most. You already know what your preferred sensory systems are based on the exercises in chapter 3. So, for example, if you are an auditory person, you are likely to be more receptive to sounds than to visual images. On the other hand, if you are a really tactile-kinesthetic person, then you are likely to be most receptive to remembering and imagining the feel of your physical experiences.

If you are primarily a tactile-kinesthetic person, then the feeling of floating will probably be more compelling than the sounds of waves washing onto the beach. If you are primarily a visual person, then the visual or pictorial image of colored lights in different parts of your body that represent physical sensations including pain will probably be most compelling. So, work your preferred sensory systems into your suggestions.

**Rule 2: State It in the Positive.** Suggestions should usually be stated in the positive as opposed to the negative. For example, you can suggest to yourself, "Every day, as I practice my self-hypnosis and read on in this book, I will notice that I am feeling better and better and more and more comfortable." This suggestion will probably be more effective than the suggestion, "I will not feel as much pain." As another example, it would probably be more effective to suggest to yourself, "I will enjoy feeling more comfort in my shoulder," than to suggest to yourself, "I will not feel pain in my shoulder."

It is generally best to avoid using the word "not," as in the form "do not," or "you will not." So, why not use "not"? The reason is that your unconscious may just forget to notice the not! By telling yourself *not* to do or experience something that you don't want, you are focusing mental attention on that very thing! While your conscious mind can make the distinction, your unconscious probably won't.

Remember this; if you are trying to avoid something, directing your attention to what you're trying to avoid, or not think about, just makes you think about it more. What you need to do is to direct your attention to something else, for instance on what you want. So, suggest to yourself what it is that you want as opposed to what it is that you *don't* want.

**Rule 3: Don't Tell Yourself to "Try"!** Don't try. Do it! The harder you *try* to do something, or *try not* to do something, the more difficult it becomes to do it or not do it. This is known as the "Law of Reverse Effect," which states that when the conscious will comes up against the imagination, the imagination always wins. What it really boils down to is this: the harder you consciously try to do something that depends on your unconscious for its execution (like falling asleep, going to the bathroom, being attracted to someone), the more likely you are to produce the *reverse effect*. For example: Try not to think of a pink elephant. The harder you try, the more difficult it becomes to get the thought out of your mind. Isn't that so? Now, try not to notice that itch on your nose. The harder you try, the stronger the itch becomes. You may not have even noticed an itch before I drew your attention to it! Now try not to scratch it. The harder you try *not* to, the greater the urge becomes.

**Rule 4: Set a Time Frame.** It is usually helpful to place a time frame on suggestions, especially when you want to suggest the lessening or end of a behavior or experience that may be worsening your pain. For example, it might be therapeutically effective to suggest to yourself, "I no longer need to clench my teeth to release tension. I now have other more effective ways of releasing tension." On the other hand, it would be less desirable to suggest to yourself something like, "I do not need to clench my teeth to release tension," or "I will not clench my teeth." This latter phrasing of the suggestion does not set any time frame. What else is wrong with these latter two suggestions?

Once again, in the above suggestions, the use of the word "not" could be misleading to the unconscious. It could possibly be interpreted by your unconscious as "I do need to clench my teeth to release tension" (minus the "not"), especially if dysfunctional clenching behavior or the idea of having no control over clenching has been imprinted in your unconscious. However, it could work to suggest, "I will no longer clench my teeth." Your unconscious will probably interpret this as meaning, "I will do the following . . ." that is, "no longer clench my teeth."

**Rule 5: Emphasize the Present Tense.** It helps to make suggestions in the present tense and to link these with suggestions of what will happen as long as these suggested changes are believable and attainable. For example:

> *I am feeling enthusiastic about exercising my new self-hypnosis coping skills, and I have more energy and feel more comfortable as I exercise these new skills. As I continue to exercise those new skills and as I learn new ones, my energy and comfort increase.*

**Rule 6: Keep It Simple and Specific (KISS).** Be as precise and specific as possible in crafting suggestions to give yourself. This will make them easier to follow. The less wordy your suggestions are, the better. Your unconscious processes not just the words, but the entire flow and feeling created by the suggestions. So be selective about your choice of words. Keep it simple and specific. When you create self-suggestions, "KISS" them! Limit the scope of your suggestions. Do not try to tackle too many problems at once. Self-hypnosis trance is a focusing mechanism. Too much at once tends to diminish focus and bring you up, out of trance.

**Rule 7: Repeat, Repeat, Repeat.** What are the three R's of self-suggestion? That's right! It really is a good idea to repeat suggestions several times, at different times, during and outside of the self-hypnosis trance state, with and without slight modification. This helps to promote the imprinting of the desired suggestions into your unconscious. I have been following this practice throughout this book. This is why I have repeated several ideas in different places using similar or slightly different wording.

# ◎ Getting Past Some Minor Problems

When you begin using self-suggestion and self-hypnosis, it's inevitable that you will encounter some minor procedural problems. These can be easily overcome. In fact, it is essential that they be overcome in order for the self-suggestions that you give yourself before or during your self-hypnosis to get through to your unconscious. Once you learn how to deal with these potential disruptors, you'll be able to deal with them easily and automatically whenever they occur.

**What If I Fall Asleep during Self-Hypnosis?** If you fall asleep during self-hypnosis, you will fall asleep. After a short while, you will wake up feeling refreshed and rested as when awakening from a needed midday nap. However, if you want to specifically give yourself a suggestion that will help you avoid falling asleep, you can read and use the following suggestion before you enter self-hypnosis:

> **Self-suggestion.** *My unconscious mind will know if I am about to fall asleep. If that happens, my unconscious will move my body slightly to alert me enough to maintain the trance state and not fall asleep.*

This is usually enough to prevent a sleep state from occurring.

**What If I Have Difficulties Settling Down and Relaxing?** All self-hypnosis and suggestion approaches can be individualized to meet your particular needs. For example, Zarren and Eimer (2001) reported about a patient of Zarren's who had a difficult time settling down to do her self-hypnosis. Her level of anxiety and stress were so high that both of her hands were in constant motion. She continued to feel stressed and in much pain. So, Zarren decided to utilize her attention to her hands as a self-hypnosis procedure, and he employed the Magnetic Hands Induction described in chapter 4 (page 71).

This patient left the office feeling very comfortable, physically and emotionally, and she said she looked forward to using her hands to help her feel good. On follow-up, she reported that her hands were helping her to deal with her stress and pain, and that there was less pain. As I described in chapter 4, you can use the Magnetic Hands Method for self-hypnosis too. It's very effective.

See how easy it is to utilize the problem by transforming it into the solution?

To summarize, if you happen to have difficulties settling down and relaxing:

1.  First become aware of the part of your body where you feel the most tension or stress.

2.  Focus your full attention on this part of your body. Don't try to change anything. Just observe and experience what you're feeling and what is going on.

3.  Then, ask your inner mind how you can use the feelings to generate an experience you can focus on and that will help you ease into self-hypnosis and self-relaxation. Wait for an idea, image, sensation, or motor response to come up.

4.  When you get a response that feels right, go with it.

5.  Concentrate on the idea, image, sensation, or motor response. Soon you will begin to notice the feelings and sensations changing. The tension will diminish, and you will feel much more relaxed.

**The Problem of Mind Wandering.** As you have been practicing self-hypnosis using your chosen method, you probably have experienced your mind wandering from time to time during your self-hypnosis experience. This is a common but minor problem that is easily handled. As soon as you realize your mind is wandering, just redirect your attention back to what you have been paying attention to (like your marble, your breathing, your laughing place, a candle flame, ocean waves, relaxing your muscles, counting, etc.). Continue to do this whenever you first become aware that you are thinking of something else. In fact, as you continue to practice your self-hypnosis, you will sharpen your concentration, and your mind will become more focused. Recall that hypnosis is, among other things, a focusing mechanism.

# ◎ How to Use Self-Suggestions with Self-Hypnosis

The first step in using self-hypnosis to change your pain experience is simply to practice entering and exiting the self-hypnosis trance state using your chosen self-induction method. Doing this repeatedly without giving yourself suggestions imprints the self-hypnosis experience in your unconscious mind.

After you have been practicing your chosen self-hypnosis method pretty consistently twice a day for a couple of weeks, you will be ready to take the second step, which is to give yourself self-suggestions *before* you enter self-hypnosis. This tells your unconscious what you want to accomplish. Then, when you are in self-hypnosis, you can relax. You don't have to worry about what to say to yourself, so you need not summon the involvement of your conscious mind. Your unconscious already knows what you want, and it can begin turning your desires into reality.

Fumbling around with wording self-suggestions during your self-hypnosis experience can lighten your self-hypnosis trance state because it brings in your conscious mind. During self-hypnosis, as much as possible, you want to give your conscious mind a needed break, and let your unconscious work for you.

There are four simple steps for giving yourself suggestions *before* entering self-hypnosis.

1. First, write down two or three (no more than four!) specific suggestions that relate to the realization of your specific change goals or to a specific dimension of experience that you want to modify.

2. Read these suggestions to yourself four to five times before you enter self-hypnosis.

3. Induce self-hypnosis. Stay in hypnosis for ten to fifteen minutes. Do not self-suggest or do self-talk. Just relax.

4. When you are ready, exit from self-hypnosis.

That's all there is to it. It's really simple and easy.

**Case Example.** Jim was a patient who reported that his chronic shoulder pain seemed to act up and get worse whenever he got angry. So, we designed several pre-hypnotic suggestions and wrote them down. Jim was instructed to transfer these suggestions to a three-by-five index card. He was told to read his self-suggestions to himself from this index card four or five times *before* he induced self-hypnosis. Then he was to put the card down and enter self-hypnosis. He was instructed *not* to talk to himself or to give himself suggestions while he was in self-hypnosis trance. He was simply to focus on being relaxed and staying in "neutral." The prehypnotic suggestions we developed for Jim were:

1. My shoulder feels comfortable when I rest it and when I move it.

2. My shoulder feels more comfortable when I control my anger.

3.   I can control my anger but still feel healthy irritation.

4.   I control my anger and remain calm and in charge when my wife criticizes me.

By reading pertinent, individualized, goal-oriented suggestions to yourself four or five times before you enter self-hypnosis, as opposed to doing self-talk *during* your self-hypnosis, you free your unconscious to do its own work during and after your self-hypnosis practice. This provides a simple way for you to communicate with your unconscious mind.

The third step in using self-hypnosis to change your pain experience is to rehearse coping strategies while you are in self-hypnosis trance. You really should feel pretty comfortable with the first two steps before you move on to this third step.

In order to minimize the involvement of your conscious mind, it helps if you prepare yourself before inducing trance. Firstly, use only one coping strategy at a time. Once you have chosen a strategy, read through it several times in the waking state before entering self-hypnosis. Then induce self-hypnosis.

When you are in self-hypnosis, you may either stay in neutral by continuing to pay attention to what you've chosen to focus on (such as your breathing, a marble, a pleasant memory, nothing at all), *or* rehearse your chosen coping strategy.

The fourth step is to use self-hypnosis to uncover ideas and gain greater insight about your hidden motivations, feelings, inner conflicts, and the negative meanings you attach to your pain. We will cover a number of ways to do this in chapter 8.

# ◎ Post-Hypnotic Suggestion

*Post-hypnotic suggestion* is the process of giving yourself instructions and suggestions before or during self-hypnosis trance about conscious or unconscious behavior you want to engage in after you emerge from self-hypnosis and re-enter the waking state. This is an important part of using self-hypnosis effectively to start and continue the process of change. Post-hypnotic suggestions can be rehearsed before or while you are in the self-hypnosis trance state. It's your choice.

**Stating Your Goals First.** It is important to tell yourself 1. your purpose for entering self-hypnosis before you enter self-hypnosis, 2. how long you want to stay in self-hypnosis, and 3. how you are going to feel after you awaken from self-hypnosis (the post-hypnotic suggestion part). For example, you can use the following format:

1.  I am going into self-hypnosis for fifteen minutes for the purpose of allowing my unconscious mind to make the adjustments necessary to help me feel [. . .] (Append your post-hypnotic goals. For example, "more comfortable, energetic, flexible, stronger," and so on.)

2a. When my deepest mind is fully aware of how much [. . .] (append your post-hypnotic goals; for example, "comfort, energy, inner strength," and so on) I have, and knows it can maintain that [. . .] for some time after I awaken myself from self-hypnosis, my eyes will blink several times and then they will open wide, and I shall come back fully alert, sound in mind, sound in body, and in control of my feelings.

Or, as an alternative awakening suggestion, you can use the following:

2b. When I emerge from my self-hypnosis at the count of five, I am going to feel [. . .] (append your post-hypnotic goals; for example, "wide awake, alert, relaxed and comfortable for some time after I awaken," or "relaxed and ready to sleep restfully throughout the night," or "motivated and full of energy").

# ◎ Instant Relaxation As an Immediately Available Coping Skill

One valuable application of post-hypnotic suggestion is the imprinting or conditioning of instant relaxation as an immediately available coping skill. Instant relaxation is a conscious or unconscious behavior you want to engage in out of self-hypnosis and in the waking state. You can use post-hypnotic suggestions to condition yourself to employ a specific instant relaxation procedure to interrupt stressful feelings whenever you first become aware of them, so that they don't escalate. This stops stress in its tracks.

By repeatedly employing instant relaxation, it becomes an automatic habit. I have already taught you instant relaxation adaptations of Zarren's Marble Method in chapters 4 and 6. I have also mentioned that you can use attention to breathing and visual fixation on an object as a method of instant relaxation. Read through the post-hypnotic suggestions below to learn exactly how to do it.

## Exercise 7.1: Post-Hypnotic Suggestions for Instant Relaxation with Attention to Breathing

The following are post-hypnotic suggestions for instant relaxation. They are derived from Zarren's Eye-Fixation Attention to Breathing Induction, which you experienced in chapter 4. Read the post-hypnotic suggestions below slowly, a few words at a time. Do this exercise two or three times.

*I'm going to teach you how to deal with momentary stressors in seconds, without closing your eyes, and without anyone knowing that you're doing it. When you are relaxed, you can't be upset, angry, or stressed, because relaxation and those feelings are emotional and physical opposites of each other. When a person begins to feel pressured, tense, or stressed, they usually feel it someplace in the upper part of their body; the chest, shoulders, neck, or in their particular area of discomfort.*

*The moment that happens to you, and you may be more aware of it more quickly from now on, look at something not too far away to focus your visual attention and take two or three very slow, deep breaths. Breathe in relaxation through your nose, and slowly release tension through your mouth. This action will bring back a part of the memory of deep relaxation and quickly melt away any feelings of pressure, tension, or stress and diminish your discomfort.*

*Now, you are sitting here reading this and probably already feeling more relaxed. Take a few very slow, deep breaths right now and feel how much more relaxed you become.*

*Did those slow, deep breaths relax you even more? If they did, they will continue to relax you instantly whenever you do this instant relaxation. It will become a good habit that you will continue to use consciously as well as automatically and unconsciously, without even thinking about it. You will find that you feel much better each time that you do it.*

How was that?

# Exercise 7.2: A Self-Healing Ritual Procedure

The following step-by-step, self-healing ritual procedure was developed by Jordan Zarren (Zarren and Eimer 2001). It associates the things that you automatically do every day without consciously thinking about them with the healing and neutral self-hypnosis state. The procedure is simple and easy to employ. All you need is your notebook to write in and your chosen self-hypnosis induction method.

In order to use this method, you must make sure to practice your self-hypnosis for ten to fifteen minutes twice a day at the same times each day. You need to write down in your notebook everything you do from the moment you wake up in the morning to the moment you go to sleep at night, in as exact detail as possible. Include your two daily self-hypnosis sessions in this daily activity schedule. You also need to write down two to three relevant suggestions to give to yourself before you induce self-hypnosis trance. Remember to "KISS" them! Make your suggestions direct and brief. That is, keep it simple and specific.

When you sit down to do your self-hypnosis, follow these four simple steps:

1.   First, read your daily activity schedule to yourself two or three times.

2.   Repeat your self-suggestions silently four or five times before starting your self-hypnosis induction. Once you enter self-hypnosis, do not self-suggest. Just relax.

3.   Induce self-hypnosis and remain in self-hypnosis for ten to fifteen minutes.

4.   When you are ready, exit self-hypnosis and continue with your activities.

You may want to use the following three self-suggestions before entering self-hypnosis or create your own.

1.   Everything that I do every day to take better care of myself, from the time I get up in the morning to the time I go to sleep at night, including doing my self-hypnosis and my sleep time, will positively increase my energy and my comfort, and diminish my discomfort.

2.   All of my healing energy will reduce and control any discomfort, and the healing energy will go to where it is needed most.

3.   Every day I feel better and more comfortable.

That's all there is to it! Let your unconscious do the rest of its good work to help you heal.

# ◎ Self-Suggestions to Promote Self-Healing

The following eight self-suggestions for empowering your unconscious mind and your self-healing are adapted from Mutter (1987). For maximum effectiveness, choose up to *four* to give yourself before entering self-hypnosis. Work with the self-suggestions you have chosen for at least several days. Then, if you wish, you can switch to another set of self-suggestions.

1.  I have survived despite all I've gone through; therefore, all of the powers that have gotten me through to this point are still with me.

2.  Should I have a flare-up, my mind will immediately remember to use one or more fitting hypnotic coping techniques to promote my self-healing.

3.  Should I have a bad dream, a flashback, or a flare-up, my mind will immediately remember that I have survived and that I will continue to improve.

4.  Because my unconscious has a sacred trust to protect me, it will cause certain healthful changes in my body by allowing me to turn, move, twist, or bend, but only within my physical capacity and not beyond it.

5.  I feel greater comfort and I stay within those limits and protect that comfort for prolonged periods of time.

6.  As I continue to heal, I am able to move, turn, twist, and bend to a greater degree, but only within my physical capacity and not beyond it.

7.  As I continue to enjoy my greater comfort, I need not fear going beyond my physical capacity and re-injuring myself.

8.  By continuing to practice my self-hypnosis, I help myself to heal.

And here are some additional suggestions to explore.

9.  My body and mind work together to strengthen my healing powers.

10. My body knows what to do to send healing energy to where it's needed most.

11. I deserve to be comfortable.

12.  I have faith in my body's healing power.

13.  Every day in every way I am getting better and better.

14.  I am on safe and solid ground.

15.  I accept myself fully and completely.

16.  I am free of old, outdated childhood needs.

17.  I am filled with positive energy.

18.  Making mistakes and then correcting them positively increases my energy and my comfort and diminishes my discomfort.

19.  Making mistakes and then correcting them releases and makes available more of my healing power to wherever it is needed most.

## Exercise 7.3:  The Mindfulness Meditation Self-Hypnosis Method

Mindfulness meditation has evolved out of the Zen Buddhist meditation tradition, and the present-day work of people such as Jon Kabat-Zinn (Kabat-Zinn 1995) and Herbert Benson (Benson 1997). The main idea is to concentrate on an idea or object and stay with it. That is what we were doing with the marble method and the attention to breathing methods.

This particular self-hypnosis method involves concentrated attention, too, but it adds another element. The object of attention is a self-suggestion, image, word, or sound that has special, positive meaning and significance and is associated with healing. Here are the steps:

1.   Sit comfortably with your feet flat on the floor, you head, neck, and back supported, and your hands resting lightly, palms-down on your thighs.

2.   Select a self-suggestion, image, word, or sound that has special meaning and significance to you. If you choose an image, word, or sound, it should be one that you associate with healing. This will serve as your mantra or object of concentration. Some potential images to choose from are: a candle flame, ocean waves, the surface of a mountain lake, forest pond, or stream, a river, the desert, the setting sun, a tree or plant, a garden, an animal, a crystal ball, or falling snow. There are many others. Some potential sounds to choose from are: the sound of ocean waves, a

running stream, a waterfall, the sounds of the forest on a summer night, a summer rain shower, chirping crickets, birds singing, or melodious singing or music. You now have the resources to choose a word or self-suggestion that meets your inner needs.

3.    Now close your eyes, breathe naturally, and begin to pay attention to your breathing without trying to change your breathing.

4.    As you continue to pay attention to your breathing, also begin to pay attention to your chosen self-suggestion, word, image, or sound. You can tie it to your breathing or not. If you choose to tie it to your breathing, continue to pay attention to your breathing, and silently say and hear, or visualize and see, your mantra or image each time you exhale. If you choose not to tie your mantra or image to your breathing, then just hear it or see it in the way that your unconscious presents it to you. As soon as you realize your mind has wandered, and you're no longer hearing or seeing your mantra or image, refocus your attention back to hearing or seeing it, whichever the case may be.

5.    When you are ready to awaken, count silently from one to five, and at five, blink your eyes, open them wide, and feel comfortable, wide awake, and yet relaxed at the same time. Your comfort will last for some time after you have completed this exercise and awakened.

## Exercise 7.4:  The Projection Self-Hypnosis Method

This step-by-step method combines several steps from previous techniques we have covered.

1.    Sit comfortably with your feet flat on the floor, your head, neck, and back supported, and your hands resting lightly, palms-down on your thighs.

2.    Now focus your visual attention on anything that literally can serve as a "projection screen"; for example, a crystal ball, a clear glass or crystal bowl filled with water, or a blank, white sheet of paper. Stare at your projection screen while you breathe normally and pay attention to your breathing without trying to change your breathing.

3.    As you continue to stare at your projection screen, allow your unconscious to bring to your conscious attention a dynamic image of an experience that it associates with pain relief and comfort. See this pain relief image in the projection screen.

Also, hear any sounds and feel any feelings associated with this experience. This pain-relief image can be something that has worked for you before, something that you think would or could work, something you use regularly, or simply a fantasy created in your imagination. When you see such an image on your projection screen, close your eyes and enter self-hypnosis.

4.   Continue to see, hear, and/or feel your pain-relief image with your eyes closed, and continue to pay attention to your breathing without trying to change your breathing. Now allow a positive healing self-suggestion or positive healing thought to come to mind. You have by now read through plenty for your unconscious to select from, or your unconscious will make up a new one. When one comes to mind, your index finger of your nondominant hand will lift. Then lower it.

5.   Mindfully meditate on (that is, concentrate on) your pain-relief image, your positive self-suggestion, and your breathing. As you do this, allow the image to change, or feel free to change it in a way that is associated with greater comfort and healing. Notice any changes that you feel in your body.

6.   Continue paying attention to the above as you direct healing energy and warmth from your hands into your body. Consciously intend this healing energy, of which there is an unlimited supply, to go wherever it's needed in your body and diminish your discomfort.

7.   Let the index finger of your nondominant hand lift up all by itself when the pain is diminished at an unconscious level. Then relax your finger.

8.   Let the index finger of your dominant hand lift up all by itself when you are consciously aware of the relief. Then relax your finger.

9.   Tell yourself that when your deepest mind knows that it can maintain the comfort you have gained and continue to process what you have learned in this exercise, your eyes will blink several times and then open wide, and you will come back fully alert, sound in mind, sound in body, and in control of your feelings.

What was that like? What did you learn? Write your insights in your notebook.

## Exercise 7.5:  Another Kinesthetic and Auditory Self-Hypnosis Method

This is another quick self-hypnosis induction method based on the eye-roll technique. I learned it from Edelstien (1981) and then adapted it. As I've outlined it in the steps below, this method is brief, simple, easy, and effective. Whenever you wish to hypnotize yourself using this method, all you need do is follow these steps:

1.    Read your one to four suggestions to yourself five times. Then put them down.

2.    Situate yourself comfortably. Look all the way upward with your eyes for about five seconds, then slowly spell the word "relax" to yourself. Imagine seeing the letters and hearing the letters as you spell the word to yourself. Straining the eyes upward, as you already have experienced, creates a tension that prepares you for entering into a trance state after you close your eyes and relax them. The word "relax" is a direct suggestion for what you expect to happen.

3.    Then take one deep breath, let it all out, let your eyelids flutter down closed, and relax your eyes and then your body. Let your eyes remain comfortably closed, without squeezing them tight, until you are ready to awaken from your self-hypnosis. Relax, breathe normally and pay attention to your breathing without trying to change your breathing.

4.    When you wish to awaken, all you need do is count backwards from three and open your eyes wide at one. Upon coming out of your self-hypnosis, as always, you will be alert, and you will feel more relaxed and comfortable for a long while after.

That's all there is to it! It's easy and can be used as an instant self-relaxation technique also. However, it should only be used as an instant self-relaxation technique when and where it is appropriate. **Never do this while driving or while doing anything where your external attention and fully alert state of mind is absolutely required.**

## Exercise 7.6:  Putting It All Together

In this section, I will summarize the main components of hypnotizing yourself out of pain that we have already covered. I am going to provide you with a seven-step hypnotic analgesia (pain relief) mental rehearsal formula. You should practice this seven-step, self-relaxation and mental rehearsal sequence at least two times a day for at least fourteen days. This will imprint the desired ideas, skills, and intended experiences in your unconscious so that you will be able to evoke the appropriate ideas and coping skills automatically and have the intended positive experiences whenever you need to. Thus, you will be prepared to handle your typical pain or a pain flare-up, should one occur.

## When to See Your Medical Doctor

First of all, you need to understand that, if the nature or quality of your pain changes in any notable way, or if its intensity increases beyond what you are used to, or have come to expect, you should see your treating physician or a competent physician as soon as possible. You will know if this is so. Trust your natural instincts and your intuition. However, if there's any doubt, see your physician for medical evaluation and appropriate treatment in any case. No new pain should go medically unevaluated and untreated. It may turn out that medical treatment is indicated.

## Seven Steps for Hypnotizing Yourself Out of Pain

Following are seven simple steps to learn, rehearse, and practice to help you get relief from your pain.

**Step 1: Waking-State Reframing.** Decatastrophize and reframe the main negative, dysfunctional thoughts associated with your negative emotional feelings in the waking state. You can't afford the luxury of languishing in negative thoughts! After you have done this, formulate one or two positive self-suggestions based on your reframing of those negative, dysfunctional thoughts. Alternatively, you may select one or two already provided for you in chapter 5. Write these self-suggestions down.

**Step 2: Record Your Purpose, Time You'll Spend In Trance, And How You Want To Feel.** You prepare for your self-hypnosis trance experience by telling yourself: 1. *why* you are entering trance, 2. *how long* you will remain in trance, and 3. *how you will feel* when you awaken from the trance state.

Write down a preparatory suggestion that approximates the following format:

> *I'm going into self-hypnosis for around twenty minutes for the purpose of [...]. When my deepest mind is fully aware of how [...] I feel, and knows it can maintain that feeling of [...] for some time after I awaken, my eyes will*

*blink several times, they will open wide, and I shall come back feeling fully alert, sound in mind, sound in body, and in control of my feelings.*

**Step 3: Consciously Choose A Hypnotic Coping Strategy.** Next, consciously choose a hypnotic coping strategy. You now have many to choose from. Go back through the exercises in chapters 5 and 6 and choose a particular deep relaxation, de-catastrophizing, direction, distraction, distortion, or dissociation strategy. After a while, you will no longer need to refer back to these chapters. The process will become automatic, one smooth flow, and you'll be able to choose the right exercise and strategy for each occasion. After you've chosen a hypnotic coping strategy, go through it and review it in your mind. Use all of your preferred senses and your active sensory imagination. Feel yourself doing it. Feel the feelings and physical sensations, see the sights, hear the sounds, smell the scents, and taste the tastes. Then, formulate one to three self-suggestions based on your strategy, or just use the one given with the exercise you have chosen from chapter 5 or 6. Write these self-suggestions down.

**Step 4: Read Your Self-Suggestions.** First, read your preparatory self-suggestion regarding *why* you're entering trance, *when* and how you will awaken, and *how you will feel* after you emerge from self-hypnosis. Then, read your coping strategy self-suggestions five times. Then, put away your self-suggestions sheet or notebook.

**Step 5: Induce the Self-Hypnosis Trance State.** Use your chosen method for inducing self-hypnosis. Trust your unconscious to monitor the time you stay in self-hypnosis trance.

**Step 6: Enjoy the Neutral Self-Hypnosis Trance State.** Don't think about giving yourself suggestions at this point. Just enjoy the experience of being in the pleasant, neutral, relaxed state of self-hypnosis. Let your unconscious work for you!

**Step 7: Further Unconscious Imprinting and Awakening.** Remain in self-hypnosis for a little while longer until you are ready to awaken. Then . . .

*When your deepest mind is fully aware of how much [your desired feeling state] you feel and knows it can maintain that feeling of [. . .] for some time after you awaken, your eyes will blink several times, and then they will open wide, and you will come back feeling fully alert, sound in mind, sound in body, and in control of your feelings.*

### Practice, Practice, Practice

Those are the seven steps for hypnotizing yourself out of pain. Your repeated practice of this sequence will imprint effective hypnotic coping skills. This will mentally condition you so that you're prepared to employ the right hypnotic coping skills automatically whenever you need to and when it's appropriate. You will be prepared to handle typical pain or pain flare-ups, or breakthrough pain. This builds your inner resources so that you can cope better and feel more comfortable more of the time.

### Waking State Suggestion

You can employ waking-state suggestion anytime to reinforce your coping resources and comfort. You can do this by writing down on an index card, and in your notebook, the self-suggestions associated with the hypnotic coping strategies that your conscious and unconscious minds have selected. Carry the index card around with you and read the self-suggestions written on the card whenever you think to do it during the course of your day. This will further imprint the coping strategies in your unconscious and make them more immediately and automatically available whenever you need them most. Also, read these self-suggestions in your notebook as your first step when you do your regular, twice or three times daily self-hypnosis sessions.

## Exercise 7.7:  GOALS for Self-Suggestions (Go On And Lick Suffering)

Do you remember your answers to the self-evaluation questions back in chapter 2? Go back to the pages in your notebook on which you recorded your responses to the questions regarding what your "key problem" was. Those questions addressed: 1. what the problem feels like; 2. what it stops you from having, doing, or feeling; 3. what it leads you to have, think, do, or feel that you would rather not; 4. what you want most that you don't have; 5. what you need to feel, do, and think to get what you want and stop getting what you don't want; and 6. what you are willing to do differently. By now, after all we've done together, you know much more about these issues. You have gained better insight, perspective, and coping skills. This chapter's final exercise will prepare you for the exercises in the next chapter, oriented to helping you solve your main inner conflicts about your pain.

Now let's employ your new learning to go on and lick suffering by setting some GOALS. Fill in the blanks below. Use your notebook. You now have another method for creating self-suggestions.


Fill in the blanks below. Write your responses in your notebook. This exercise will help you clarify your goals and create pertinent self-suggestions.


For me, the problem is _(what?)____. What I want is _(what?)____. I need _(what?)____ to get what I want. To the degree that I want _(what?)____, I will _(do what?)____.

The pain feels like _(what?)_____. Its positive opposite is _(what?)_____. How I want to feel is _____. So, from now on, whenever I feel, see, or hear _(what?)_____, I will think, do, and feel _(what instead?)_____. I will feel _(what?)_____when I do, think, and/or feel _(what?)_____.

**Case Example.** Sara had migraine headaches that were stopping her from getting to work consistently. This is how Sara filled in the blanks:

For me, the problem is *the stress at work.* What I want is *to be treated fairly.* I need *to be more assertive* to get what I want. To the degree that I want *this*, I will *practice speaking up for my rights.*

The pain feels like *a hammer.* Its positive opposite is *peace and quiet.* How I want to feel is *strong and safe.* So, from now on, whenever I feel, see, or hear *my boss yelling at me or criticizing me*, I will *tell him that I will not let him treat me so abusively.* I will feel *stronger and better about myself* when I do *that.*

When Sara was able to respond differently to her boss, she began to feel stronger. Incidentally, her boss's behavior also began to change in response to the change in Sara's behavior. During Sara's self-hypnosis, she suggested to herself that entering self-hypnosis helped her "dip into the healing peace and quiet, the reserves of strength" she needed. She also visualized and rehearsed assertive responses to her boss before she dipped into self-hypnosis trance. The result was a notable decrease in how much her migraine headaches "hammered" her and an improvement in her functionality.

# EIGHT

## Solve Inner Conflicts about Your Pain

*The unconscious mind is aware of body functions and dysfunctions; therefore, we can utilize the power of the unconscious as a diagnostic instrument . . . Hypnosis may be used to explore the source of a physical problem when usual diagnostic techniques have failed to reveal it.*

**—Charles Mutter, M.D.**

*Conflict* means disharmony, strife, contention, controversy, friction, argument, dissension, dissonance, division, and confrontation. Conflict unfortunately tends to be a given when you have chronic, persistent pain. That is because chronic pain robs you of your ability to fulfill the role obligations you used to take for granted and used to perform regularly and consistently. Conflict creates stress, and stress worsens chronic pain.

For example, your employer may want you back at work. You may want to be able to go back to work, but you cannot. Your family members may want the "old you" back, but the old you may no longer exist in the same form. You may want the old you back, and that person may want to come back, but the reality of the new you with the pain may not be capable of accommodating the old you. All of this precipitates inner conflict, and this creates more stress and more pain.

It is natural to seek to avoid or escape from pain of all types. That is what this book is all about. However, it is sometimes necessary to confront and deal with the source of the pain before you can make it go away. This is often the case with emotionally painful thoughts and feelings.

# ◎ The Problem of Repression

It is natural for the mind to employ defense mechanisms that are designed to keep painful thoughts and feelings away, out of conscious awareness. However, this can create a problem. The problem is that when certain thoughts and feelings are *suppressed* (deliberately kept out of conscious awareness), or *repressed* (kept from ever becoming conscious in the first place), they actually can stand in the way of pain relief.

There is an old saying which states *that which you resist tends to persist.* So, if you consciously or unconsciously resist dealing with your painful or conflictual emotional feelings and thoughts related to your physical pain, they will persist and continue to create trouble for you. Undealt with, they actually can prevent you from feeling and getting better, or even feeling that you deserve to feel better! They can block you from effectively using pain coping skills. They block you by keeping you stuck, as if you are frozen in the past.

Hypnotizing yourself out of pain and feeling better involve changing your present and creating a different, brighter future. In order to do so, you have to identify and change outdated, negative ideas and meanings that are holding you back and inhibiting you from healing.

Because they are loaded with pain, many of these negative ideas and meanings are suppressed or repressed. However, from the depths of your inner mind, they affect how you feel physically and emotionally and how you behave. They create dilemmas that lead you to feel "damned if you do, and damned if you don't."

For example, if you try to do something that you have been unable to do because of your pain and you find that you can't accomplish it (such as returning to work or fulfilling family role obligations like you used to), you may suffer the indignity of feeling ineffective. There are worse things, but if this leads you to try too hard, you may re-injure yourself and worsen your pain. On the other hand, if you don't try, you may feel like a failure or worse. You may feel like you're caught between a rock and a hard place. You may feel trapped. This is not unusual. I've been there myself.

Repressed, or unconscious, negative ideas and feelings can make you feel hopeless about ever being able to change anything or gain any measure of control over your symptoms and how you handle your pain. The more negative ideas, meanings, and feelings that are stuffed inside, suppressed and repressed, the more internal pressure there is likely to be. The more internal pressure there is, the more everyday hassles can seem overwhelming. That is because they just add to the pressure that is already there. So, the main sources of this internal pressure have to be dealt with. The repressed thoughts and feelings and inner conflicts need to faced and resolved.

If you are in the habit of dwelling on negative thoughts and feelings that you're conscious of (such as the belief that you're a disappointment, or feelings of guilt or anger), you may never get to solve the real problems lurking beneath the surface. In a nutshell, the real problems are the negative beliefs, attitudes, and feelings that you are not conscious of, or are only dimly aware of, or feel hopeless about addressing in a positive way.

In this chapter, we are going to explore a number of hypnotic methods for honing in on and reframing (changing how you think about) these unconscious or subconscious negative beliefs, attitudes, and feelings that block you from healing and feeling better.

The use of hypnotic methods to uncover, explore, and change hidden, suppressed, or repressed feelings and meanings that affect your symptoms and block your healing is called *hypno-analysis*.

## ◎ Not Every Method Is for Everyone

As I have said before, not every method is for everyone. That's why I give you choices. The purpose of the exercises in this chapter is to help you uncover, process, resolve, and get past the unconscious ideas and feelings associated with your pain that have outlived their usefulness and that perpetuate continued suffering. Confronting old, buried, or repressed hurts can bring up pain. Therefore, you may feel that you want to consult with a licensed mental-health professional (a licensed clinical psychologist, clinical social worker, or psychiatrist who does hypnotherapy) to help you deal with this type of pain.

# ◎ You Will Take Care of Yourself

Let me reassure you that you will know if and when you need the help of a licensed health professional to help you deal with your problem. In each exercise to follow, you will be asking your unconscious, inner mind for permission—that is, if it's okay to proceed. If you don't get the go ahead, then don't go ahead! Because you will be able to choose the hypno-analysis methods that feel right for you to employ on your own, the methods you choose will work and will be appropriate for you to use as I guide you through each process. Listen to your unconscious, and listen to your body. It will not lie to you.

» You will only go as far as you are ready to go and no further.

» Your unconscious will continue to protect you by making sure that you go no further than you can handle.

» You will be able to stop at any time if you encounter material that your inner wisdom tells you is better processed with the assistance of a licensed mental-health professional.

At the beginning of some exercises, you will be given one or two questions to consider that will enable you to determine if the exercise is appropriate for you. If an exercise isn't right for you, skip it and pick up on the material following it.

## Exercise 8.1: The Beginning of Your Pain

Often, a controlled review of the incident that you believe is responsible for your present condition can help you to gain greater control over your symptoms and even diminish those symptoms. This is the premise that the following exercise is based on.

### *Instructions*

If you believe you know the event that was responsible for the initial onset of your pain problem, you can employ the following hypnotic review technique. If you do not believe you know, you can skip this exercise, or you can focus on a past experience when your pain took a turn for the worse. If the experience you choose to focus on was associated with a great deal of hurt, and you feel uncomfortable reviewing it on your own, then you can select another, more manageable experience. If you feel that you would be better off not doing this exercise alone, then don't proceed with this exercise. In that case, consider seeking competent therapeutic supervision, guidance, and support, as can be provided by a qualified, licensed therapist well-trained in hypnosis. If you are going to do this exercise now, follow the steps below.

*As with all of the hypnotic exercises in this book, when you are situated comfortably and absorbed in your self-hypnosis experience, each time you turn a page, you will become more absorbed and go deeper into self-hypnosis.*

1.  First, situate yourself comfortably as you have done in the earlier exercises in which you read yourself into self-hypnosis. Then, begin reading the script below very, very slowly, a few words at a time. You will read yourself into self-hypnosis, as you have already done many times before by now. With each word that you read and each breath that you take, you will move further and deeper into self-hypnosis.

2.  After you have finished doing the exercise through reading and have returned to an awake state, put this book down, pick up your notebook, and write down any relevant information you have learned or discovered. Then, proceed to step three.

3.  Induce self-hypnosis in your preferred way and do the exercise again with your eyes closed. When you have finished doing the reviews of the incident you've selected with your eyes closed, return once again to an awake state, and write down any additional relevant information you have learned or discovered in your personal notebook.

*Take a few slow, deep breaths, breathing in relaxation and exhaling tension. Then breathe normally and pay attention to your breathing without trying to change your breathing.*

*In a few moments you are going to do a controlled review of the incident that you believe is originally responsible for your present condition or of a past incident when your pain took a turn for the worse. This can help you to gain greater control over your symptoms and even diminish those symptoms. Each time you review the experience that you believe caused your present condition, you will find that some aspects of the experience become more vivid, but you will also notice less pain at the moment when the pain began, at the moment it became worse, or when it became too important. In fact, when you have completed this mental review exercise, you will also notice that the current physical and emotional pain is diminished.*

*When you are ready, go back in your mind to that moment in time just before your pain began, got worse, or became too important. What are you doing? Where are you? Whom are you with? Notice all of these things, and see, hear, and feel what is happening. Be aware of your body movements and position. Does anyone say anything that seems important, or that makes an impression? What are you thinking? What are you feeling at the moment that the injury occurs? At the moment that the pain begins or gets worse? At the moment that the pain becomes too important?*

*As you review this experience, the pain may change in some way. Continue through whatever is occurring. Review what is happening and what you're experiencing up to that point in time when you know that the experience is over and that you are safe. Go back through and review this experience a second time.*

*After you have gone through the experience a second time, I would like you to review that experience again, but this time in reverse. Starting at the point in time when you know that the experience is over and that you are safe, go backwards in time to the moment in time just before your pain began, became worse, or became too important. After you have done this once, do it again. Good.*

*When you have completed your reviews, and when your deepest mind knows that it can maintain the comfort you have gained and also continue to process in a nonintrusive way what you have learned in this exercise, blink your eyes, open them wide, and come back fully alert, sound in mind, sound in body, and in control of your feelings.*

What was that like? How do you feel now compared to before this trance experience? Write any insights you've gained in your notebook.

## Exercise 8.2: Mentally Scanning and Reframing Past Hurts

This procedure is used when you are not sure of any particular incident associated with the onset of your pain problem. It is adapted from Jordan Zarren's Silent Abreaction Procedure (Zarren and Eimer 2001). It will enable you to safely scan past hurts and work through some of the past experiences that may have contributed to the continuation of your pain experience. To begin, situate yourself comfortably in a safe and tranquil place where you will not be bothered or disturbed. Then start reading.

*As you read these words very slowly, a few words at a time, you will enter self-hypnosis. Each time you turn a page, you will become more absorbed and go even deeper into self-hypnosis. As you continue to read these words, I am going to guide you to do some exploration of the past. You* will be able to explore in your own mind visually, kinesthetically, and emotionally, considering those things that have occurred that you need to put closure on, that you need to work through, and that you need to feel comfortable about from now on. These are things that you need to leave in the past in order to be able to change your experience of the present. By leaving these things in the past where they belong, you free yourself from unnecessary discomfort in the present and imprint the positive expectation of having a more comfortable experience in the future. You have already had the opportunity to learn and practice relaxation procedures, which have helped reduce your experience of discomfort. You feel more in charge of yourself. As you read on and continue to go deeper into relaxation, allow yourself to feel more and more comfortable. When you feel that you have reached the greatest level of comfort that you can reach today, let your nondominant index finger lift up all by itself to verify that you've reached that level of comfort. Then lower your finger. Good. Now I'm going to ask that you count backwards slowly from 30 down to 1. With each number that you count, you will go deeper and deeper into relaxation and hypnosis. You'll find yourself not only going deeper into self-relaxation and self-hypnosis, but you'll also find yourself moving rather quickly back into the past. You will find yourself moving back in time to the earliest time that you can remember when you felt hurt, when you felt extreme emotional and physical pain, when you felt great fear, or felt a great deal of guilt. And when you are there, you will encounter those experiences armed and protected with all of the present-day knowledge and coping skills that you have now, as a more mature you.   In the safety of where you are situated right now, you can silently work through those experiences and change their meaning so that they no longer have any validity or influence on your present and future feelings. If that feels okay to you, your nondominant index finger will lift up to verify that it feels okay. After you finger lifts, lower your finger, thank your unconscious, and continue reading. However, if your finger does not lift, then stop here, skip the rest of this exercise, and continue reading the material that begins after this exercise. If this happens, it's perfectly all right. Your unconscious exists to protect you and keep you safe. It will only let you experience what you're ready to safely experience.   If your inner mind gave you the okay to continue now, you are going to be able to encounter these experiences and silently work through the meaning that those experiences imprinted in your unconscious mind then. You are going to change those meanings now so that they no longer have any validity or influence on your present and future feelings and experiences. So, as long as you have the "go ahead," begin by slowly reading the numbers below. Let yourself go and find yourself going back in time, back into the past, as you go deeper and deeper into relaxation and hypnosis. 30 ... 29 ... 28 ... 27 ... 26 ... 25 ... 24 ...

*23…22…21…20…19…18…17…16…15…14…13…12…11…10*
*…9…8…7…6…5…4…3…2…and…1.*

*Now that we've reached the number 1, you can start the process of exploring those past experiences and begin to work through them, resolving them, and changing their meaning. Remember, time has no meaning when you're in hypnosis. You can process hours of real time in minutes while you are in trance. So, go ahead and process what's happened. And when you've reached the present once again, after you have worked through all of those pertinent experiences, just let your nondominant index finger lift up to signal that you've completed the process. Then relax your finger. This whole process may take anywhere from ten minutes to thirty minutes, depending on how many hurts you encounter and deal with and how intense those experiences are. When you have completed this task of exploration from the earliest time you remember to the present, your nondominant index finger will lift up again to inform you that you have completed this process. Then lower your finger. Now you've explored all of the things you can remember from the past to the present that have had some effect upon and influence upon the continuing chronic discomfort that you've been experiencing. As a result of this exploration, you can now leave behind you, as only a memory, those things that contributed to the problem then, but which are no longer happening or relevant anymore now. Because you can leave those old, outdated, memories behind, back there in the past, you can begin now, in the present, to experience a greater sense of comfort. You can begin now, in the present, to experience a greater sense of resolution, a greater sense of optimism, and a greater sense of closure on those things that may have contributed to your discomfort problem. Those things no longer need affect you now. You are going to realize that you have pretty much freed yourself from most of that emotional overlay that had contributed to the ongoing intensity of your discomfort and pain. And from now on, every time you do your own self-hypnosis and relaxation, without having to go back into the past, you are going to be able to recognize and experience a greater sense of freedom, a greater sense of comfort, and a greater sense of well-being. Now let yourself be relaxed. And when your deepest mind knows that it can maintain the comfort you have gained and continue to process in a nonintrusive way any leftover remnants from the past and add to your new, positive learning experience, blink your eyes, open them wide, and come back fully alert, sound in mind, sound in body, and in control of your feelings.*

What was that like? How do you feel now compared to before this trance experience? Write any additional insights in your notebook.

# Exercise 8.3: Zarren's Scrolling Blackboard Technique

This procedure is adapted from Jordan Zarren's gentle, hypnotic uncovering method called the Scrolling Blackboard Technique (Zarren and Eimer 2001). It provides a way to clean your emotional slate by erasing old hurts.

*As you read these words very slowly, a few words at a time, you will enter self-hypnosis. With each word you read and each time you turn a page, you will become more absorbed, and go deeper into self-hypnosis. As you continue to read these words, I am going to guide you to do some exploration of the past. You have already learned how to enter a comfortable level of relaxation and hypnosis. So, put yourself back into relaxation now and experience the healing power of the Neutral and Healing Place. This is the place where there are no pressures, tensions, or discomforts. The place where you can begin to erase the problems of the past and leave them behind, where they can do no harm.*

*Do you remember when you were in school and each classroom had a blackboard on which you could write with chalk and erase what you wrote when you wanted to? Can you imagine such a place now, with a blackboard that you will be able to write on in your imagination? When you have that blackboard fixed in your mind, your nondominant index finger will lift up all by itself to verify this. After it lifts up, lower it so that you can continue. Good. Now imagine that this is a modern blackboard that has an automatic scrolling feature. It will allow you to write a lot, and it will scroll to produce more space as you need it. Do you have the scrolling feature on your blackboard? Your index finger will lift up and then relax when you do. Great.*

*Now take that chalk that is on the blackboard ledge, go back as far as you can in your mind, and begin to write everything that you can remember that happened to you that was hurtful, harmful, fearful, uncomfortable, or emotionally unpleasant. Include your physical hurts as well as your emotional hurts. Be as detailed as you can be. Include people, places, and things.*

*Don't be concerned about how long it will take for this task to be accomplished. During hypnosis, time is very flexible. What seems like a long time to you could be only a short time during hypnosis, and what seems like a short time could really cover a long period in your life. Be as complete as you can, and take as much time as you need. Notice that as you finish writing with your chalk on a section of the blackboard, it automatically scrolls up, creating a clean panel available for your writing.*

*When you have written everything that you possibly can, right up to the present time, again permit your index finger to lift up and then relax. Good. Now, look at the blackboard and note that it is scrolling back to the beginning. Check over everything that you have written and make sure that you haven't left anything out. If you need to add anything, extra space will appear for you to fill in what you want to. When you have finished checking your work, your index finger will lift up and relax to verify this. Good.*

*Now, take the eraser that is on the shelf and, starting with the most recent thing that you have written, begin to erase it. Notice that the blackboard scroll function is working in reverse. Erase every bit of chalk writing that you see. Wipe the slate clean. Remove all of the things that you wrote that caused hurt, whether it was physical or emotional. Wipe it out. Remove it. Leave no trace. Take whatever time you need and erase every bit of it. Don't leave anything. When you have wiped the slate clean, go back and remove any remnants that may be left. When you have completed this task, your index finger will lift up to verify this. Now relax it.*

*Just continue to sit for a while feeling very relaxed, very clean, and very comfortable. And, when your deepest mind knows that it can maintain the comfort you have gained and continue to process in a nonintrusive, beneficial way any remnants, blink your eyes, open them wide, and come back fully alert, sound in mind, sound in body, and in control of your feelings.*

How do you feel now compared to before this trance experience? You may benefit by adding this scrolling blackboard to one of the two daily self-hypnosis sessions that are already part of your daily ritual. This addition will not add much time to your self-relaxation session because the purpose is to deal with any leftover hurts that come to your mind. Your level of discomfort will be significantly reduced because the buildup of hurt that has, up until now, been responsible for some of your emotional overlay will be dissipated.

Do this for a week and then reevaluate how you feel. After a week of adding this procedure to one of your two daily self-hypnosis sessions, you will be aware that you feel lighter, more energetic, and stronger, as if you are carrying less emotional baggage with you. You can add this procedure to one of your two daily self-hypnosis sessions again, at any time in the future, if there happens to be a cumulative buildup of emotional stress that needs to be erased. By doing so, you will lighten your burdens and ease your pain.

# ◎ The Seven Emotional Keys to Persistent Pain

By this point in your journey through this book, you understand why, despite your continued efforts, the pain may still persist. You may also be more aware of the negative emotional feelings (like anxiety, fear, depression, anger, guilt) that are brought up by and exacerbate your pain. These feeling states are overlaid on top of the physical pain, and that is why I call them a negative emotional overlay. This emotional overlay constitutes the *suffering* element of chronic, persistent pain. Quoting Dabney Ewin from the foreword, "Pure pain without a psychic overlay is generally quite tolerable and is often of value in limiting overexertion."

You understand that your use of coping strategies helps you deal with the stress associated with persistent pain and helps you reduce the negative emotional overlay to manageable proportions. You understand that pain is influenced by multiple factors; physical, medical, biological, mental, psychological, emotional, and social. Among these factors are the unconscious, negative ideas and meanings that have outlived their usefulness. You understand that all of these factors affect how pain signals are processed by your central nervous system, which in turn affects how much pain you feel.

Back in the 1960s, David Cheek and Leslie LeCron (Cheek and LeCron 1968) developed a hypnotic tool called the "seven keys" to understand the main types of unconscious negative ideas and meanings and emotional factors that could give rise to or maintain persistent pain states. They and many subsequent therapists have found the seven keys to be helpful for uncovering the specific meanings and experiences *underlying* a patient's persistent pain state, much in the way that a detective uncovers clues to solve a case. The seven keys tool has proven especially helpful in situations where no identifiable physical cause for the pain can be isolated, and the severity of the pain seems to be out of proportion to the magnitude of the objective physical findings. However, as you shall learn, these keys operate in almost every case where pain persists indefinitely.

The seven emotional keys to persistent pain are: conflicts, "organ language," motivational factors, past experiences, attachments, self-punishment, and self-suggestions. Each emotional key opens the door to understanding an unconscious issue that could be having a profound influence on your pain experience. Therefore, it's important that each of these doors are opened so that you can have a look inside.

Please keep in mind that these emotional keys are not independent issues. They are separate, but interrelated. Each "door" ultimately leads to the same "inner room": your inner room inside your unconscious mind. Our objective, with your permission, is to have a look around inside that room. There may be things inside that room that need to be cleaned out. Once the room is cleaned out, the air inside will be a lot fresher and less stuffy. Also, once your inner room is cleaned out, there will be less clutter inside. When there is less clutter inside, you will be able to move around a lot easier.

# ◎ Communicating with Your Inner Mind

In order to find out which emotional keys open which doors, you need a way of communicating with your unconscious or inner mind. Just asking yourself in a conscious, awake state which of the keys are operative is not as effective as asking yourself the right questions while you are in self-hypnosis. That is because, when you are in self-hypnosis, the doorway to your unconscious opens and you can exchange with your unconscious the information needed to make the changes you want to make; namely, to diminish your pain, alleviate your suffering, and gain greater control over your symptoms.

The best way to communicate with your unconscious while you are in self-hypnosis is a way that helps you to become more focused and absorbed in your self-hypnosis trance state so that the doorway to your unconscious opens wider. Recall my earlier statement that doing self-talk and giving yourself self-suggestions while you're in hypnosis can lighten your hypnotic state. That is the opposite of what you want to do. To uncover unconscious information that will help you solve aspects of your pain problem, you need to be adequately focused and absorbed in self-hypnosis.

## Ideomotor Finger Signalling

Cheek and LeCron (1968) also developed a method for communicating with the unconscious. This method is called *ideomotor finger signalling* and you already have been using ideomotor finger signals throughout this book. Whenever I have asked you to allow the index finger on your nondominant hand to lift up all by itself when you were having a particular experience, and then lower or relax that finger, that was ideomotor finger signalling. Wasn't that easy? Ideomotor finger signalling enables you to stay focused and absorbed in trance as you communicate with your unconscious. It sharpens your concentration, increases your absorption, promotes deeper relaxation, and heightens your receptivity and responsiveness to your body's meaningful communications in your body's own language.

Cheek and LeCron (1968) taught us that the unconscious, or inner mind, communicates its feelings all the time with unconscious movements. For example, we may nod our head or smile without being aware of it when something feels "yes," or shake our head "no" or frown or tense up without being aware of it when something does not feel right or feels "no." This is called ideomotor behavior, which means unconscious ideas ("ideo") transformed into motor actions ("motor").

Ideomotor finger signalling means transforming an unconscious idea into a finger signal. We are going to focus on signals for the following three ideas: 1. yes, 2. no, and 3. I don't know or I'm not ready to answer that question yet. Let's go ahead and set up this ideomotor finger signalling system.

### Setting Up the System

Begin by sitting comfortably with your head and back well supported, and your feet flat on the floor. Rest your hands with the palms facing down either on your thighs, on the table in front of you, or on the arm rests of the chair. Now focus on your hands.

1.  If you ask yourself a question and the answer feels like "yes," your *index finger* on your *nondominant* hand will slowly rise up all by itself to let you know that the answer is "yes." Say "yes, yes, yes" to yourself and raise your nondominant index finger. Then lower it. Good. Now you know which finger is your "yes" finger.

2.  If you ask yourself a question and the answer feels like"no," your *middle finger* on your *nondominant* hand will slowly rise up all by itself to let you know that the answer is "no." Say "no, no, no" to yourself and raise your nondominant middle finger. Then lower it. Good. Now you know which finger is your "no" finger.

3.  If you ask yourself a question and the answer feels like "I don't know," or "I'm not ready to answer that yet," or "I'm not ready yet," your *thumb* on your *nondominant* hand will slowly rise up all by itself to let you know that the answer is "I don't know." Say "I don't know, I don't know, I don't know" to yourself and raise your nondominant thumb.

Then lower it. Now say, "I'm not ready yet, I'm not ready yet, I'm not ready yet," and raise that same thumb again. Then lower it. Good. Now you know which finger is your "I don't know" and "I'm not ready to answer yet" finger.

You now have your ideomotor finger signalling system in place. While it may be obvious why you need the "yes" and "no" signals, the third signal may be more confusing. Of course, if you don't know an answer, you'll need to indicate that. But raising your thumb also can mean that you're not ready to pursue the answer to a particular question. Having this signal available allows your unconscious to easily protect you from information that you're not ready for yet. This signal is your way of opting out and staying safe.

## Exercise 8.4: Exploring the "Seven Keys" with Ideomotor Finger Signals.

The following exercise is adapted from the work of David Cheek (Cheek 1994; Cheek and LeCron 1968; Rossi and Cheek 1988), Leslie LeCron (LeCron 1964), and Dabney Ewin (Ewin 1986, 1992). It is based on the following set of basic assumptions.

At one time in the past, your now chronic pain was acute and functional. It helped you to survive some physical insult or threat to your body. Some time after the original insult or threat occurred, that acute pain began to feel *too important*. It persisted beyond the point where you would have expected it to go away. But it didn't go away, and its persistence felt inexplicable. You naturally began to wonder if it would ever go away. A lot of anxiety probably resulted. This anxiety, along with any other intense emotional feelings you were experiencing at that time, became associated with the pain.

The pain as a message from your body signifying that something is wrong, along with these intense emotional feelings, became fixed or, as I have used the term, imprinted in your unconscious along with certain negative and dysfunctional ideas. As the pain continued and didn't go away, it created stress, and this stress intensified your negative emotional experience and reinforced the strength of your negative and dysfunctional ideas.

You are now tired of being in pain. You want to feel better. You want to get well. In order for you to feel better, these old thoughts, feelings, and experiences need to be uncovered and reviewed. The subconscious negative ideas and meanings that have outlived their usefulness have to be reframed so that you can start to think and feel differently about what happened then and what is happening now. You need to come to the point where you can accept the belief that you no longer need all of the pain. You need to believe on both a conscious and unconscious level that, at one time, your pain served an important signalling function that assured your survival. At that time in the past, you needed the pain to survive. However, you did survive. You are alive, and you no longer need the pain, or as much pain, to survive now.

The following exercise will enable you to accomplish this reframing process if you're ready. If you are not ready, your unconscious will let you know. In that case, you can skip ahead to the next chapter. Or, if you want to proceed with this exploration, you should consider seeking the services of a qualified, licensed therapist who is skilled and experienced in the use of clinical hypnosis and hypno-analysis.

For the following exercise, get comfortably seated as you were in the previous exercises in which you read yourself into self-hypnosis. Your hands should be resting with the palms facing down, either on a table on either side of your book, on your thighs, or on the chair's arm rests. As before, your book should be propped up in front of you.

Begin by taking several slow deep breaths. Then, breathe normally and pay attention to your breathing without trying to control or change your breathing as you read through and experience this exercise.

*As in previous exercises, read slowly, a few words at a time. As you read the words in this exercise and concentrate on the fingers on your nondominant hand, with each and every word you read and each and every breath you take, you will go further and deeper into self-hypnosis with your eyes open. Your eyes will remain open throughout this entire exercise so that you can continue to read and respond to the instructions and suggestions. Your dominant hand will remain ready to lift up to turn the page each time you need to do so to read on. After that hand turns the page, it will return to the position it was in before and remain ready to lift up again to turn the next page when you are ready to do so. Each time you turn a page, you will become more absorbed and go even deeper into self-hypnosis.*

*In this exercise, I'm going to guide you in searching your inner mind for answers to certain questions about the psychological factors that could be maintaining your pain. Concentrate on the fingers on your nondominant hand and let them do the talking. After you ask your inner mind each question, wait for a finger to lift up all by itself, and then lower it. As you do this, you will go deeper and deeper into self-hypnosis.*

*Later, when you complete this exercise and exit from self-hypnosis, write your thoughts about what you've learned in your notebook so that you can refer back to them at a later time.*

*The very first thing you need to do is to ask your inner mind, your unconscious, if it feels okay to do this. Using your fingers to answer, ask yourself the following question:* **Is it all right for me to know what psychological or emotional factors are maintaining my pain or worsening it?** *If any finger other than your "yes" finger lifts up, it indicates that your inner mind has reservations. In that case, do not proceed further with this exploration of your unconscious unless you are doing so with an experienced, licensed therapist who is qualified to use hypnosis for purposes of hypnotic uncovering and hypno-analysis. If you are working alone, skip this exercise, and move on to Exercise 8.5. However, if your "yes" finger lifted up, your unconscious has given you the go ahead. So, proceed with the exercise.*

*The first emotional key is conflict. It refers to internal or external disagreement and disharmony. This is created when there are competing values, needs, or demands within a person or between one person and others. Conflicts create stress, and stress worsens pain. Using your fingers to answer, ask yourself:* **Is my pain associated in some way with a conflict of any kind or a problem that I have making some sort of decision?** *If your "no" or "I don't know/I'm not ready yet" finger lifts, go on to the next key. If your "yes" finger lifts, ask your unconscious to give you some indication about the nature of the conflict. Just wait for thoughts, images, and feelings to come to mind. When you feel that your unconscious has brought to mind the thoughts, images, and feelings that make clear the nature of this conflict, your "yes" finger will lift up to verify that this feels right. However, if your "yes" finger does not lift up within a reasonable period of time, go on to the next key.*

*The solution to your conflict, whatever it is, is to* **make a decision**. *So tell yourself:* **When I think about my pain, I realize I have choices. I can make a decision to do something and choose what that "something" is or simply do nothing.**

*The second key is organ language. "Organ language" means that sometimes a negative emotional feeling is talked about as if it were a physical problem. For example, we've all heard people say things like, "He's a pain in the neck'" or "It's a headache'" or "I can't stomach this'" or "It's eating me up'" or "It's holding me back." In fact, emotional feelings are converted into or experienced as physical feelings much of the time. Using your fingers to answer, ask yourself:* **Is my pain associated in some way with organ language of any kind?** *If your "no" or "I don't know/I'm not ready yet" finger lifts, go on to the next key. If your "yes" finger lifts, ask your unconscious to give you some indication about the nature of this organ* *language and how it perpetuates your pain. Just think of the question and wait for thoughts, images, and feelings to come to mind. When you feel that your unconscious has brought to mind the thoughts, images, and feelings that make clear the nature of this organ language, your "yes" finger will lift up to verify that this feels right. However, if your "yes" finger does not lift up within a reasonable period of time, go on to the next key.*

*The solution to organ language is to* **develop the habit of being conscious of the words you use to describe your feelings about things and develop the habit of challenging and disputing self-defeating and dysfunctional thoughts and self-talk. So tell yourself: I remember to be conscious of the words I use to describe how I feel about things. I no longer need to accept every thought as valid or true.**

*Proceed in the same way for each of the remaining keys. If you get a "no" or "I don't know/I'm not ready yet" response to your first question, "Is my pain in some way related to that key?", go on to the next key. If you get a "yes" response, ask your unconscious for information about the nature of that key and how it is related to your pain. However, if your unconscious doesn't bring up this information within a reasonable period of time, move on to the next key.*

*The third key is motivation. Motivation refers to the underlying, unconscious reasons why a person unconsciously assumes particular ways of coping with pain. Motivation refers to unconscious needs that are being met by the way the person copes. Sometimes these needs conflict with other needs, such as when the need to be strong and independent conflicts with the need to be taken care of.*

*Using your fingers to answer, ask your self:* **Is my pain associated in some way with an unconscious need or motive of any kind? Is it a need or motive I am unaware of consciously?** *If you get a "yes," explore this further. Ask yourself what the motive or motives are. If you get a "no" or "I don't know/I'm not ready yet," proceed on to the next key.*

*The solution to motivation is to keep your priorities straight, and stop confusing what you want with what you need. So tell yourself:* **I no longer confuse what I want with what I need to survive. I keep my priorities straight. I continue to maintain healthy desires, but I no longer need to be demanding.**

*The fourth key is past experience. Using your fingers to answer, ask your self:* **Is my pain associated in some way to a past experience of any kind?** *If you get a "no," go on to the next key. If you get a "yes," ask your self:* **Is it all right for me to know what this past experience was?** *If you get a "no" or "I don't know/I'm not ready yet," go on to the next key. If you get a "yes," proceed as follows. Focus on the pain sensations and your emotional feelings about them. Let these sensations and feelings become a bridge into your past. Travel over that bridge to the very first time you ever experienced these sensations and feelings; to the very first moment that you felt that this pain was really serious, really important. As you count backward from 10 to 0, you will travel backward to an earlier time, to another place. At the count of 0, you will arrive at the situation that first produced these sensations and feelings. When you have arrived there, let your "yes" finger lift up to verify that you are there. Then relax that finger. Begin counting now ... 10 ... 9 ... 8 ... 7 ... 6 ... 5 ... 4 ... 3 ... 2 ... 1 ... 0.*

*In the safety of the present, review what was happening at that time. When you begin your review, let your "yes" finger lift up to signal that you have begun your review. Then lower your finger. Your thumb will lift up and then relax when you have completed your review of the incident.*

*Your pain was the best way your body knew to protect itself from further injury at that time. Therefore, the pain was very important back then. The pain let you know that you needed to get help. It let you know that something was going on that you needed to pay attention to, something that needed to be taken care of. So, the pain was necessary then. It helped you survive. And you did survive. You are here today reading this book to learn how you can hypnotize yourself out of pain and learn to live with less pain and greater comfort.*

*The next step is to ask your inner mind:* **Using my fingers, please let me know if you feel that this pain has already served its purpose.** *Wait for a finger signal. Note which finger lifts up. No matter which finger lifts, ask your inner mind:* **Do you know now that we have other ways to protect me from further injury, and we have different ways to manage and diminish the pain?**

*If your "yes" finger lifts, list all of these alternative ways in your mind. Say them out loud. Later you can write your list down in your notebook. However, if your "no" or "I don't know/I'm not ready yet" finger lifts, ask your inner mind:* **What prevents you from knowing that we now have other ways to protect me from further injury and different ways to handle and lessen the pain?**

*Just think of the question and wait for some thoughts, images, or feelings to come to mind. When your unconscious brings to mind some thoughts, images, or feelings that clarify its reluctance to acknowledge that you have resources now that you didn't have then, your "yes" finger will lift up to verify this. Then lower the finger and go on to the next question. However, if your "yes" finger does not lift up within a reasonable period of time, go on to the next question anyhow.*

**Now that we have other ways to prevent further injury, and lessen pain, do we still need all of this pain to protect me from further injury?** *A "yes" answer requires further exploration, which often uncovers fears and concerns that may have once been valid but are no longer valid now. If you get a "yes" answer, ask your inner mind:* **Are there any fears or concerns that you have that continue to make the pain very important?** *If you get a "yes," ask the following question and then wait for an answer:* **Please make me consciously aware of what these fears or concerns are.**

*Note what comes up. Later you can write down what's important to remember in your notebook. If you become aware of some major concerns that have a realistic or medical basis, then you may need to stop this procedure here and deal with them. In that case, you can resume this procedure at a later date, once these fears and concerns are realistically and appropriately addressed. However, if you got a "no" or "I don't know/I'm not ready yet," then ask:* **Since we don't need all of this pain anymore, and I now know different ways to handle it, diminish it, and get rid of it, would it be all right to let at least some of it go?**

*A "yes" answer calls for turning off or diminishing the pain first at an unconscious level and then letting the change become conscious. However, a "no" answer calls for asking your inner mind what purpose the pain still serves. Ask:* **What purpose does the pain still serve?** *Wait for an answer to come to mind and then ask:* **Knowing that this pain still serves an important purpose, do I still need all of it to serve that purpose?** *If you get a "yes" response, stop here and skip to Exercise 8.5. You will need the help of a trained therapist to proceed further with this particular exploration if you wish to do so. However, if you get a "no" response, ask:* **Knowing that all of the pain is no longer needed, would it be all right to diminish it to a more comfortable and tolerable level? Would it be all right to let some of it go?** *A "yes" answer calls for turning off or diminishing the pain first at an unconscious level and then letting the change become conscious. However again, if you get a "no" or "I don't know/I'm not ready yet" answer, stop here and skip to Exercise 8.5.*

*If you wish to proceed further with this exploration, you should obtain the assistance of a trained therapist.*

*If your unconscious has signalled that it feels all right to be more comfortable, you can turn off or at least turn down the pain.* **Ask your inner mind to turn off the pain on an inner unconscious level and to signal with your "yes" finger when this has been accomplished. Wait for your "yes" finger to lift up and then relax it.**

*It will take a short while longer before you become consciously aware of the comfort. When you do, consciously lift up your "yes" finger and then relax it. Then:* **Ask your unconscious for a commitment to maintain this comfort for a specified time period. Let your "yes" finger lift up when this is accomplished. How long is the commitment for?** *When your deepest mind knows that it can maintain the comfort you have gained and continue to process what you have learned in this exercise, your eyes will blink several times and then open wide, and you will come back fully alert, sound in mind, sound in body, and in control of your feelings.*

**If You Can Make It Get Worse, You Can Make It Get Better!** Dabney Ewin (Ewin 1986, 1992) has pointed out that if the pain temporarily becomes worse soon after doing this exercise, there is no need to worry. If this happens, it indicates that you have been able to gain control of the pain and make it worse, and therefore, you can also make it better whenever you choose. He suggests that, if this is the case, you should ask your inner mind whether it would like to cut the pain in half right now? If you get the "yes" signal, follow the procedure described above for turning it down. Then, ask your inner mind: **Would it be all right for me to have one minute completely free of pain, realizing it's better to live without pain than to live with pain?** If you get a "yes," ask your inner mind to turn the pain off for one minute. Now, if you can do this for one minute, then you can do it whenever you are ready for two, four, six, eight minutes, a half hour, an hour, and so on. **You gradually can gain more and more control over the pain with the cooperation of your inner mind. You own this control. You can also choose when to exercise this greater control. Save it for when you need it the most.**

What I mean is that when you have physical impairment and disability, there are times when it is functional to feel more pain so that you do not overdo activities and end up re-injuring yourself. Then there are other times when there is no need for the same level of pain.

The solution to past experience is to tell yourself and believe in your deepest mind the following: **I am a survivor. I no longer need all this pain to survive. I remember that it is better to live without pain than to live with pain.**

**Re-enter Self-Hypnosis and Work through the Remaining Keys.** Now go back into self-hypnosis by reading the questions on the remaining three keys below, very slowly, a few words at a time. You will quickly become absorbed once again in the self-hypnosis experience and find yourself once again completely engaged in the remainder of this exercise.

*The fifth key is attachment. Using your fingers to answer, ask yourself:* **Is my pain associated in some way with an identification I have with someone from the past or the present? A person to whom I am, or was, very attached who had a similar type of pain or who suffered from some other type of severe pain?**

*If you get a "no," go on to the next key. If you get a "yes," ask yourself:* **Is it all right for me to know who that person is or was?** *If you get a "no" or "I don't know/I'm not ready yet," go on to the next key. If you get a "yes," that person's identity will come to you. When you become consciously aware of who that person was, ask yourself:* **Would [person's name] have wanted me to suffer like he or she did?** *I'm sure your "no" finger will lift up. Now move on to the next key.*

*The solution to attachment is to realize that if you won't get well for yourself, perhaps you'll do it for those you love and who love you. So ask yourself:* **Don't I know that I need to be free of all unnecessary pain, if not for my own sake, then for the sake of those who love me? Would [person to whom you're attached] want me to suffer like he or she did?**

*The sixth key is self-punishment. Using your fingers to answer, ask yourself:* **Is self-punishment involved in my pain problem? Have I been consciously or unconsciously continuing to punish myself with this pain?**

*If you get a "no" or "I don't know/I'm not ready yet," proceed on to the next key. If you get a "yes," ask yourself:* **Does it have to do with something that I did that I feel guilty for?** *If you get a "no" or "I don't know/I'm not ready yet," ask:* **Does it have to do with something that I feel guilty for not doing?** *If you get a "no" or "I don't know/I'm not ready yet," go on to the next key. If you get a "yes" to either of the above questions, ask your inner mind:* **Would it be all right for me to know consciously what it is?**

*If you get a "no" or "I don't know/I'm not ready yet," move on to the next key. In that case, your unconscious is not ready to make this information conscious to you yet. However, if you get a "yes," ask your unconscious the following question and wait for an answer to come up:* **Please make me aware of the crime for which I have been punished.** *Note what comes up. Later you can write down what's important to remember in your notebook. However, the solution to self-punishment is to suggest the following to your inner mind:* **Everyone is entitled to a good defense, even me. It is unjust for me to serve as my own jury and judge. I've served enough time in pain. I've been punished more than enough to pay in full for any old crimes I may have been guilty of committing. I forgive myself for all of my past mistakes. I also forgive others whom I have been angry at. If I have been angry at God, I forgive God, too.**

*The seventh key is* **Self-suggestion.** *Using your fingers to answer, ask yourself:* **Has someone ever said anything to me that might be causing much of the pain? Is there some suggestion working? Some idea that somehow got imprinted in my subconscious mind?**

*If you get a "no" or "I don't know/I'm not ready yet," you have completed your ideomotor review of the seven keys. However, if you get a "yes," ask yourself:* **Would it be all right for me to know consciously what was said?**

*If you get a "no" or "I don't know/I'm not ready yet," you have completed your ideomotor review of the seven keys. You have gone as far as you can take yourself on your own, and you have done well! Commend yourself. If you wish, you can always consider seeking the assistance of a licensed, trained therapist who uses hypnosis to explore further.*

*If you get a "yes," that it's all right for you to know consciously what the imprinted suggestion is, then ask your unconscious to make you aware of the suggestion. Just think of it and wait for thoughts, images, and feelings to come to mind. When you feel that your unconscious has brought to mind the thoughts, images, and feelings that make clear the nature of this specific suggestion, your "yes" finger will lift up to verify that this feels "yes."*

*The solution to self-suggestion is to realize that you can give yourself permission to be free of all negative ideas and meanings that have outlived their usefulness, because they are all invalid now. You will feel more comfortable when you do this.*

## Solutions through Positive Opposites

As you have seen, these seven keys provide the basis for generating some very powerful and moving self-suggestions for reframing, decatastrophizing, self-directing, and inner healing based on each of the key's "positive opposites" (the daydreams that translate into relief). These self-suggestions provide solutions to the problems posed by each key, and they are summarized below.

**Conflict.** When I think about my pain, I realize I have choices. I can make a decision to do something and choose what that "something" is, or simply do nothing.

**Organ Language.** I remember to be conscious of the words I use to describe how I feel about things. I no longer need to accept every thought as valid or true.

**Motivation.** I no longer confuse what I want with what I need to survive. I keep my priorities straight. I continue to maintain healthy desires, but I no longer need to be demanding.

**Past Experience.** I am a survivor. I no longer need all this pain to survive. I remember that it is better to live without pain than to live with pain.

**Attachment.** I know that I need to be free of all unnecessary pain, if not for my own sake, then for the sake of those who love me. Would [person to whom you're attached] want me to suffer like he or she did?

**Self-Punishment.** Everyone is entitled to a good defense, even me. It is unjust for me to serve as my own jury and judge. I've served enough time in pain. I've been punished more than enough to pay in full for any old crimes I may have been guilty of committing. I forgive myself for all of my past mistakes. I also forgive others whom I have been angry at. If I have been angry at God, I forgive God, too.

**Self-suggestion.** I can now give myself permission to be free of all negative ideas and meanings that have outlived their usefulness.

## Exercise 8.5:  Ego State Therapy

The following exercise is based on the pioneering work of Dr. John Watkins and Helen Watkins, two innovative and compassionate clinical psychologists who are the father and mother of Ego State Therapy (Watkins and Watkins 1997). It provides another way of uncovering and solving inner emotional conflicts or issues that may be maintaining your persistent pain.

We all talk to ourselves. We all have mixed emotions about things. Different parts of us feel differently about things. So at times, different parts of us may be in conflict. We are all aware that sometimes one part of us may want one thing, while another part of us doesn't want it and may want something else. For example, one part of you may want surgery, but another part of you won't let you have surgery. One part of you may want to give up, while other parts of you will not let this happen.

These different parts of us, these different aspects or facets of our personality, provide a system of checks and balances in our mind. For example, one part of you may feel that you're guilty of a crime and deserve punishment, while other, wiser parts of you (possibly, your internal defense attorney?) may feel that you cannot be your own jury and judge.

Most of the time these inner aspects or parts of your personality are silent, and hence, you are unaware of their existence until an issue comes up that requires their inner voices to be heard in the form of self-talk, feelings, or pain. For example, can you recall the last time your "inner critic" told you that you're not good enough?

With our tool of self-hypnosis, you can communicate with these inner voices now. Every member of this inner family of your "selves" is of course affected by the physical pain in your body, because they are all a part of you. Using self-hypnosis, you can communicate with those parts of you that have something to say about or do with your pain. In fact, it actually is possible to talk with the part of you that originally accepted the pain or first had the pain, and the part of you that is holding onto the pain currently. Using the step-by-step method below, you can negotiate with those parts of you, those inner voices, or "ego states" as Watkins and Watkins call them, to come up with a more comfortable solution for all parts of you. Now try the script below.

> *Read this script in the same way that you have read other hypnotic scripts in this book—very slowly, a few words at a time. After you have read fifteen to twenty-five words, you will enter self-hypnosis. Your eyes will remain open so that you can continue reading, and with each word you read and each breath you take, you become more and more focused and absorbed as you go deeper and deeper into self-hypnosis. Hypnosis is a focusing mechanism. Each time you turn a page, you become more focused and absorbed and go even deeper into self-hypnosis.*

> *Now, kindly walk down the set of twenty plushly carpeted stairs with the highly polished wood railing that lies before you into a private conference room at the bottom of the stairs. If you cannot walk down stairs, there is*

*a working elevator available for your use. If you don't like elevators, there is even a handicapped accessible, ADA-approved ramp that goes down to the lower floor so that you can get down there comfortably. Now, enter the conference room at the bottom of the stairs. In this conference room, you can hold an internal board meeting with your inner voices, inner selves, or as Jack and Helen Watkins put it, your different ego states. These are all different names for the same thing; the different parts of you affected by this pain, all of whom have something to contribute toward finding a more comfortable solution that is acceptable to all parts of you.*

*First have a seat at the conference table in the conference room. When you are situated comfortably, ask the part of you that originally accepted or took in the pain to please come into the room and kindly announce his or her presence. When he or she walks through the door or appears, your nondominant index finger will lift up and then relax to verify this. Thank that part of you for coming forward, and invite him or her to sit down at the table. Then ask that part what his or her name is, or what he or she would like to be called. Ask how old you were when he or she first appeared and first took in your pain. Ask what was happening at the time to you that caused that part of you to come into being and accept your pain. Commend and thank that part of you for sharing this information, also for coming into being to help you, and for having the courage and strength to take in and hold the pain.*

*Now ask that part of you if it is largely responsible for holding onto your pain currently. If it responds that it is, thank him or her for sharing this information with you and for coming forward to talk with you. Invite this part to kindly remain so that he or she can continue to participate in this inner conference and help in finding a continuing solution that is more comfortable than the pain was.*

*If this part responds that it is not largely responsible for holding onto your pain now, ask it if it knows the part of you that is. If it does, thank him or her for sharing this information with you and for coming forward to talk with you. Invite this part to kindly remain so that he or she can continue to participate in this inner conference and help in finding a continuing solution that is more comfortable than the pain was.*

*If it responds that it does not know which part of you is largely responsible for holding onto your pain currently, thank him or her for talking with you. Invite him or her to remain so that he or she can continue to participate in this inner conference and help in finding a continuing solution that is more comfortable than the pain was.*

*Then ask the part of you that is responsible for holding onto your current pain to please come forward. Wait for him or her to walk through the door into the room, or appear. When he or she enters the room, your nondominant index finger will lift up and then relax to verify this. Thank that part for coming in, invite him or her to have a seat at the conference table, and ask what his or her name is. Invite this part to kindly stay and participate in the conference.*

*Ask the part how old you were when he or she first appeared and first took on the pain. Ask what was happening at that time that motivated him or her to come into being, take on the pain, and continue to hold onto it up through the present. Commend and thank that part of you for coming into being to help you, and for having the courage and strength to take on the pain, and continue to hold onto it. Ask this part if he or she is willing to participate in coming up with a continuing solution that is more comfortable than the pain has been for all concerned. If the part answers "No," you will need to be creative to find a way to convince it to say "Yes." Negotiate.*

*Ask the part what his or her current purpose or goal is. If the goal it states is obviously commendable, express your appreciation and thank it for taking such pain to serve your greater needs for survival. If the goal or purpose it states sounds destructive, you will need to be creative and reframe this goal so that it can be thought of instead as being motivated by good intentions; that is, to help you survive. Then express your appreciation and thanks. Remind this part of you that you have survived. Tell him or her that now there are other, more comfortable ways for everyone involved to help all of you continue to survive. Assure this part of you that if he or she agrees to adopt a different method to help you continue to survive, then he or she will continue to survive and thrive as a valued member of your inner family of selves.*

*Tell this part of you that, if he or she would be willing to permit you to take the pain away, you will nurture him or her and continue to do so. Tell him or her:*

*"The pain is from the past, but I'm from your present and future. The pain was needed then to help us survive. It worked—we did survive. I can handle our pain now. I have read this book, and now I have many helpful coping skills and strategies that I didn't have before. I will be able to continue to use these coping skills to handle and diminish the pain, if you let me."*

*Ask this part what he or she needs and wants. Assure the part that his or her needs will NOT go unmet, because you will find the best ways to continue meeting these needs if he or she lets go of the pain and gives it back to you to handle from now on. Your job is to use all of your creative intelligence to persuade that part of you to believe in the advantages of allowing you to be more comfortable from now on. Negotiate.*

*Check in with all of the other parts of you. Invite everyone to participate in finding an alternative way to meet the above part's current needs in a way that is acceptable to everyone and that doesn't interfere with anyone else's needs being met.*

*If the part's needs are a remnant from the past, ask every part of you that may have something to contribute to come into the room, have a seat at the table, and make themselves heard. Work with everyone in the room to come up with an acceptable way to update that original part's needs. Make sure to obtain that part's agreement that the solution you all come up with is acceptable.*

*Check out and mentally rehearse several alternative ways in your inner mind for meeting everyone's needs in a more comfortable way. When you have come up with a way that feels right, check in with all parts of you, all of your "inner voices," all of your inner selves, to make sure that there are no objections to that way. If any part does voice objections, explore what these objections are and negotiate an acceptable compromise. If no part objects, ask for a commitment from all parts of you to use the way that you all have chosen for a week or two to see how it works. Agree to reconvene at the end of that period to reevaluate how things have gone.*

*Thank everyone for participating in this inner conference. Assure everyone that from now on, no one's voice will be ignored because they are all part of you; that every part of you depends on you to survive, and that you depend on them and care about all of them. As the Three Musketeers said, "One for all, and all for one."*

*Now just continue to sit for a short while longer, feeling very relaxed and very comfortable. And, when your deepest mind knows that this conference today is successfully concluded and that the comfortable solutions you have agreed to have been accepted and can be implemented, you can awaken from your self-hypnosis in one of two ways: you can choose to walk back up those twenty stairs, and when you reach the top of the stairs, blink your eyes, open them wide, and come back fully alert, sound in mind, sound in body, and in control of your feelings; or you can choose not to walk back up those stairs and just blink your eyes, open them wide, and come back fully alert, sound in mind, sound in body, and in control of your feelings.*

## Exercise 8.6:   The Inner Conference Table Technique

This exercise takes you straight into your own inner conference room. It is another strategy adapted from John Watkins and Helen Watkins (1997). First, as in the previous exercises, you induce self-hypnosis. Then, as before, you walk down a set of twenty plushly carpeted stairs to an inner conference room. When you enter this room, you see an oblong conference table with chairs around it. You take a seat facing the door.

*You sit watching the door. Wait for someone else to walk into the room who might know something important about your pain and who wants to be heard. When someone appears, invite him or her in to have a seat at the table. Ask him or her their name. If no one appears after you've been waiting for a while, that's okay, too. No one may want to make an appearance at this time. If that happens, you can use this room as a place to think, relax, or meditate, and when you're ready to emerge from your room, you can do so, walking back up the twenty steps and awakening from your self-hypnosis. You can simply do this exercise at another time.*

*However, when someone does enter the room who has something important to contribute, proceed as follows together. Ask that someone who he or she is and what his or her name is. Then, ask what he or she knows about your pain. Also, ask what he or she knows about how you can become more comfortable and about how you can get well. Ask what you need to do to live without pain or live with less pain.*

*When you and this person or being have finished talking or are ready to have someone else join your conference, ask for everyone else involved in your pain problem to kindly enter the room and have a seat at the table. Ask everyone who enters to introduce themselves. Ask each individual or "ego state" what he or she knows about your pain, what he or she knows about how you can become more comfortable, and about how you can get well. Ask: "What must I start doing so that I can live without pain, or with less pain?"*

*Make sure that, as you talk with the different ego states, you work toward finding solutions that serve everyone's, that is, every ego state's needs. Remember that everyone who shows up to participate in your inner conference is there for a reason. Also, be aware that there may be some silent ego states who, for their own good reasons, have chosen to observe and not participate. You want to make sure that the solutions you come up with are acceptable to all. Therefore, you want to give everyone the opportunity to make themselves heard, if they wish.*

*You are also in an appropriate place now to call upon "wise beings" or inner advisors who can help you find greater comfort. In this special, safe place, you can call up anyone, living or dead, with whom you feel a special attachment or connection. This may be someone you know or knew to whom you were attached in some important way, or even a famous person from the past whom you have never met, but with whom you have a special affinity; someone whom you respect and like. My personal inner advisors are . . . Wait a minute! I cannot divulge who they are, nor should you. It's best to keep their identities to yourself. I and my inner advisors have agreed to maintain a confidential relationship so that we can speak freely. So can you!*

*Now just continue to sit for a short while longer, feeling very relaxed and very comfortable. And, when your deepest mind knows that this conference today is successfully concluded and that the comfortable solutions you have agreed to have been accepted and can be implemented, you can awaken from your self-hypnosis in one of two ways: you can choose to walk back up those twenty stairs, and when you reach the top of the stairs, blink your eyes, open them wide, and come back fully alert, sound in mind, sound in body, and in control of your feelings; or you can choose not to walk back up those stairs and just blink your eyes, open them wide, and come back fully alert, sound in mind, sound in body, and in control of your feelings.*

# ◎ A Prayer for Healing

At the time of writing this, the Jewish High Holy Days (Rosh Hashanah and Yom Kippur), I came across a prayer that moved me, that captures the spirit of appealing to a Higher Power for the resolution of conflict and the attainment of inner peace and healing. I end the chapter with this prayer for these priceless blessings (Stern 1996, 407).

O Source of peace, lead us to peace, a peace profound and true; lead us to a healing, to mastery of all that drives us to war within ourselves and with others. May our deeds inscribe us in the Book of life and blessing, righteousness and peace! O Source of peace, bless us with peace. Amen.

# NINE

## Become AWARE and Find Your Inner Balance

*God, grant me the serenity to accept the things I cannot change, the courage to change the things I can, and the wisdom to know the difference.*

**—Reinhold Niebuhr**

*Life is short, and it's up to you to make it sweet.*

**—Sadie Delany**

All of us who have chronic pain in a major way know that it tends to change our personality. Over time, the continued struggle with pain tends to zap your energy and strength. Life is harder and more stressful when persistent pain is a central part of it. The hurt of days spent in pain adds up and collects its toll by persistently eroding your resilience and hardiness. This is the reality of the chronic pain experience.

For many of us, at times it feels as if managing pain is a full-time job. The relentless interference of pain can lead to remarkable levels of distress and disability in one's social and occupational functioning. Unfortunately, these changes also affect one's outlook on life and one's personality functioning. Such is the reality of the chronic pain experience.

Fortunately, now there are things you can do to cope better and improve your quality of life with a little help from self-hypnosis.

## ◎ Be AWARE and Find Your Balance

I want to end this positive book on a positive note by summarizing a helpful set of suggestions for finding a functional balance between the opposing forces of acceptance and change. To *accept* means to concede to, agree to, tolerate, endure, allow, receive, or even welcome and embrace as opposed to reject, refuse, renounce, or deny. To *change* means to alter, modify, convert, transform, correct, shift, or vary. Coping with chronic pain effectively, which means *as comfortably as possible*, necessitates finding a functional balance between these two opposite forces.

The roadmap or outline I shall provide is called AWARE. It is built on a basic idea that I have emphasized throughout this book. That is the idea that to be *aware* need not mean being obsessed or preoccupied with negatives. Healthy awareness is a necessary precondition to changing something. You need to know (become aware of) what needs to be changed in order to develop a strategy for changing it. So goes the old adage, "If you don't know where you want to go, how are you going to get there?"

Awareness also goes along with the idea of acceptance. It's clear to me that when you have chronic pain due to a permanent physical injury, impairment, or disease, the best philosophical course to follow is one of acceptance. You need not like that you have it, but if you don't accept it and accept yourself even though you have it, how can you take constructive action? Constructive action and effective coping depend on acknowledging what is, even if you don't like it. However, if you can find a way to embrace and love your pain adversary at an appropriate level, you will find that it's easier to cope with it and be happy. Either way, you need to accept and love yourself.

Gerald Jampolsky, M.D., a psychiatrist and originator of an approach to self-healing called "attitudinal healing" (Jampolsky 1979), has coined the phrase that "love is letting go of fear." I think that this is definitely true when it comes to coping with chronic pain. Equipped with the self-hypnosis tools you have studied, you are now more capable of letting go of the paralyzing fear that can make pain worse and of having a healthier relationship with your pain.

Please understand that awareness, acceptance, and loving do not mean not changing. On the contrary, rejecting and refusing to acknowledge and accept reality, or denial, is what can block you from initiating and continuing the process of genuine and healthy change.

Linehan (1993) has wisely pointed out that the key to effective therapy for facilitating change with regard to chronic problems is balancing actively *striving for change* (a traditionally Western European and American philosophy and approach) and *inwardly searching for acceptance* (a traditionally Eastern and Asian philosophy). So . . .

# ◎ AWARE Self-Suggestions

The acronym "AWARE" stands for **A**ccept the pain, **W**atch your experience, **A**ct functionally, **R**emove yourself from pain, and **E**xpect the best. The AWARE self-suggestions are:

## I Accept the Pain

1. I understand the puzzle of pain.

2. I no longer need to continue to fight all the time.

3. The pain is becoming less important.

4. I compare my qualities and behaviors only to those of myself.

5. I forgive myself and no longer need to keep punishing myself.

## I Watch the Pattern of the Pain

1. I notice what's working in my life.

2. I evaluate my pain, my life, and my coping strategies.

3. I notice where, when, and how I feel comfortable.

4. I use self-hypnosis to solve my inner conflicts about my pain.

5. "Hurt" does not necessarily mean "harm."

6. I separate "necessary" from "unnecessary" pain.

## I Act Functionally despite Having Pain

1. I optimize the control I have in managing my discomfort.

2. I motivate myself by doing things I am interested in and enjoy.

3. I evaluate my priorities and schedule my time.

4. I use pain coping skills.

5. I direct my own behavior and take charge.

6. I direct myself to experience pleasure.

7. I interrupt dysfunctional feelings, thoughts, and behaviors.

8. I balance *accepting* and *watching* my experience with *distancing* or *dissociating* myself from unnecessary pain.

9. I identify with positive role models.

10. I increase my rest time without feeling guilty if I get a flare-up.

11. I negotiate support from others and ask for help when I need it.

## I Remove Myself from Unnecessary Pain

1. I do my self-relaxation and self-hypnosis regularly.

2. I avoid stressful situations and don't let myself become too stressed.

3. I distract myself from discomfort.

4. I employ my attention flexibly.

5. I use my most engaging and absorbing sensory memory systems.

6. I regularly make deposits in and withdrawals from my positive memory bank.

7. I control unnecessary pain by distorting and transforming it.

8. When it's appropriate, I disconnect and detach myself from unnecessary pain.

9. I direct unnecessary pain to go away.

## I Expect the Best

1.  I am open to choices and opportunities for improving the quality of my life.

2.  I remain optimistic, flexible, and open to change.

3.  I build motivation by finding good reasons to change.

4.  I reframe dysfunctional beliefs.

5.  I dispute negative, irrational, and dysfunctional thoughts.

6.  I help myself into a positive frame of mind with self-hypnosis.

7.  I use positive self-suggestion and coping self-statements.

All of these self-suggestions are part of your new "hypnotize yourself out of pain now" program. They can be employed in the waking state and before entering self-hypnosis to continue the process of positive self-change on an unconscious level. When you employ these self-suggestions in the waking state, they serve as positive affirmations and help you direct your own behavior and experience.

# ◎ You Can Do It!

Yes. You *can* do it. You have all the tools you need to continue hypnotizing yourself out of pain *now*. I hope that you have found reading this book a valuable, enjoyable adventure and a helpful and comfortable experience. I wish you the best on your continuing journey.

# TEN

## How To Select A Qualified Clinical Hypnosis Practitioner

*Once you've established the credentials, it's important that you feel comfortable with the psychologist, [or other licensed health professional] since your treatment will involve working together as a team. A good rapport with your psychologist [or other licensed health professional] is critical. Choose a psychologist [or other licensed health professional] with whom you feel comfortable and at ease."*

**—American Psychological Association (1997)**

If you decide that you want to see a clinical hypnosis practitioner, how should you go about finding someone who is qualified? You can begin by inquiring with your local psychological, medical, dental, or other health-care discipline society in the area where you live, you can ask your physician for a referral, or you can ask others with similar problems as yours for a referral. If you use the Yellow Pages, you will need to do a lot more screening on the telephone of the prospective professional.

## ◎ Do Your Homework

Your best bet is to find a licensed health professional who is properly trained and with whom you feel comfortable. First of all, consider the following questions:

1.  How much does the person know about chronic pain? Does he or she specialize in the use of hypnosis for pain management?

2.  How much experience does the person have working with people who have chronic pain?

3.  What types of chronic pain problems has the individual helped other people with? Has he or she helped other people with similar pain problems as yours?

4.  If the person is a licensed mental-health professional and psychotherapist (like a psychiatrist, clinical psychologist, or clinical social worker), you also will want to know whether he or she has expertise treating people who suffer from the related problems of anxiety, depression, and the effects of trauma.

5.  Make sure you feel comfortable talking with the person. If you do not, look elsewhere!

**Consumer Beware.** Unfortunately, the practice of hypnosis is not regulated by most states as is the practice of other healing arts. Therefore, in most states, clinicians and therapists who use hypnosis are not licensed in hypnosis. The implications of this are that there is little or no control over who can call themselves a "certified" hypnotherapist, or "clinical hypnotist," and hang out a shingle! So beware of unscrupulous practitioners and quacks.

**Screening a Practitioner's Qualifications.** Careful questioning on the telephone can help you avoid wasting time and money with the wrong person. Whoever you choose to work with should be licensed by the state in a major health-care field such as medicine, dentistry, psychiatry, psychology, clinical social work, mental-health counseling, marriage and family therapy, pastoral counseling, or nursing.

Find out what academic degrees qualify the person to practice as a licensed health professional. Where did the individual earn his or her degrees? Was it from a recognized, nationally and state accredited college or university? Is the person a member of the major professional organizations in his or her field (for example, the American Medical Association, American Dental Association, American Psychological Association, American Psychiatric Association, National Association of Social Workers, etc.)? Is he or she a member of the American Society of Clinical Hypnosis? This is the only nationally recognized organization in the United States whose membership is restricted to state-licensed health-care professionals with appropriate training and experience in hypnosis. If you have doubts about the person's qualifications, keep looking.

**The American Society of Clinical Hypnosis (ASCH).** This is the largest national professional association of licensed health-care and mental-health professionals who use hypnosis in treating a wide range of medical, dental, and psychological conditions. Membership in ASCH is limited to clinicians who meet all of their state and national licensure or certification requirements for their particular health profession. Those requirements vary for each state, but are based on similar standards of appropriate formal education, specialized training, examinations, and supervised experience.

ASCH publishes a well-regarded, peer-reviewed journal and provides training for health professionals and students. For full membership, one must have an appropriate advanced academic degree in one's profession. In addition, a member must have a requisite number of hours of training in hypnosis provided by an approved provider of such training. A period of documented, supervised experience in the applications of hypnosis is also required, as is documented continuing education that is updated and checked every two to three years.

Professionals who are accepted for membership in ASCH sign an agreement to abide by the rules of ethics of this society. But remember that membership in this organisation is no guarantee of competence!

**Certification by the American Society of Clinical Hypnosis.** There is another important credential that aids in the identification of a qualified hypnosis practitioner. The American Society of Clinical Hypnosis (ASCH) makes available a voluntary credentialing process in clinical hypnosis. It recognizes professionals who have obtained advanced training and who have extensive experience in the use of hypnosis in their professional practices. There are two levels of such certification. The entry level is called "Certification," and the higher credential is called "Approved Consultant."

ASCH certification is distinct from that offered by other programs in that it insures that the certified individual is a bona fide licensed health professional who is recognized by his or her peers as qualified by virtue of training to provide clinical hypnosis services in a safe and responsible way. However, it does not verify competence! Verification of certification on either level may be obtained by contacting the ASCH national office (address is given below). The clinician may also have the certificate displayed in his or her office.

**Board Certification in Hypnosis.** The highest level of recognition of competence in the practice of clinical hypnosis is board certification by one of the four constituent bodies of the American Board of Clinical Hypnosis. These separate but interlinked boards are: the American Board of Medical Hypnosis (ABMH), the American Board of Psychological Hypnosis (ABPH), the American Board of Hypnosis in Dentistry (ABHD), and the American Hypnosis Board for Clinical Social Work (AHBSW). Each of these boards verifies competence to practice clinical hypnosis within one's primary health-care discipline by thorough evaluation of credentials, training, and experience, and rigorous oral and written competency examination. Becoming a Board Certified Diplomate in clinical hypnosis with any of these four boards is recognized as the highest credentialing achievement available for the practicing clinician in hypnosis.

Application for these board certifications is a voluntary, nonstatutory process. Not all licensed health professionals who use hypnosis regularly and who have adequate qualifications to sit for board certification choose to pursue the rigorous requirements for the specialty board hypnosis certificate in their discipline.

# ◎ Where to Obtain Further Information

You may obtain information about clinical hypnosis as well the names of qualified clinical hypnosis practitioners in your area by contacting the following organizations:

1.  The American Society of Clinical Hypnosis 140 N. Bloomingdale Road, Bloomingdale, IL 60108 Tel: 630-980-4740 Fax: 630-351-8490 E-mail: info@asch.netWebsite: http://www.asch.net

2.  American Psychological Association, Division 30, Society for Psychological Hypnosis 750 First Street, N.E., Washington D.C. 20002Tel: 202-336-6013 Website: http://www.apa.org/divisions/div30

3.  HypnosisHelpCenter.net P.O. Box 6, Huntingdon Valley, PA 19006 Tel: 215-947-7867 Website: http://www.hypnosishelpcenter.net

Remember that from the standpoint of seeking out a competent, ethical, clinical practitioner, your best bet is to seek a licensed health professional who has certification by the American Society of Clinical Hypnosis (ASCH) and basic, intermediate, and advanced training in clinical hypnosis offered by the American Society of Clinical Hypnosis (ASCH). The way to bet on getting the best clinical hypnosis practitioner for you is to select a well-trained, licensed, ethical health practitioner who specializes in the use of hypnosis for chronic pain management and who has a lot of experience working with people who have chronic pain.

However, I cannot emphasize enough the importance of feeling comfortable with the person. Technical competence, training, advanced degrees, authorship of publications, fame, and affiliations with recognized professional organizations are important, but if you find that you're dealing with someone with whom you feel uncomfortable, then you are not likely to accomplish anything worthwhile with that person. You should remember that the practice of clinical hypnosis and hypnotherapy is all about empathy, listening, feeling, seeing, hearing, and understanding. The person you choose to go to should be empathic and good at listening to you, seeing you, and feeling with you. If you don't feel understood, accepted, and heard, how is the practitioner going to help you change negative meanings and dysfunctional ideas?

# ◎ Contact Information

If you'd like to contact me for more information, please do so at:

Bruce N. Eimer, Ph.D., Alternative Behavior Associates and HypnosisHelpCenter.net, P.O. Box 6, Huntingdon Valley, PA 19006 Telephone: 215-947-STOP (7867) E-mail: dr.eimer@hypnosishelpcenter.net or dr.eimer1@comcast.net

Website: www.hypnosishelpcenter.net

I welcome your communication for the purpose of sharing your experiences, insights, challenges, and successes using the self-hypnosis pain-coping tools in this book.

If you've found this book to be informative, helpful, supportive, understanding, realistic, and enjoyable, then keep it handy so that you can refer back to it often. It is best to read it several times. Think of this book as your personal expert reference source for information on using self-hypnosis for pain management. The more you refer to *Hypnotize Yourself Out of Pain Now!*, the more powerful and user-friendly this pain-relief program will become for you.

# Recommended Further Reading

Affinito, M. G. 1999. *When to Forgive: A Healing Guide.* Oakland, CA: New Harbinger Publications.

Alberti, R. E., and M. L. Emmons. 2001. *Your Perfect Right: Assertiveness and Equality in Your Life and Relationships,* 8th ed. San Luis Obispo, CA: Impact Publishers.

Alman, B. M., and P. Lambrou. 1992. *Self-Hypnosis: The Complete Manual for Health and Self-Change,* 2nd ed. New York: Brunner/Mazel.

Bowers, K. S. 1983. *Hypnosis for the Seriously Curious.* New York: W. W. Norton.

Burns, D. D. 1980. *Feeling Good: The New Mood Therapy.* New York: William Morrow Co.

Catalano, E. M., and K. M. Hardin. 1996. *The Chronic Pain Control Workbook: A Step-by-Step Guide for Coping with and Overcoming Pain,* 2nd ed. Oakland, CA: New Harbinger Publications.

Caudill, M. A. 1995. *Managing Pain before It Manages You.* New York: Guilford Press.

Childre, D., and H. Martin. 1999. *The Heartmath Solution.* San Francisco, CA: HarperCollins.

Davich, V. N. 1998. *The Best Guide to Meditation.* Los Angeles, CA: Renaissance Books.

DeGood, D. E. 1997. *The Headache and Neck Pain Workbook: An Integrated Mind and Body Program.* Oakland, CA: New Harbinger Publications.

Drum, D. 1999. *The Chronic Pain Sourcebook.* Los Angeles, CA: Lowell House.

Duckro, P. N., W. D. Richardson, and J. E. Marchall. 1995. *Taking Control of Your Headaches: How to Get the Treatment You Need.* New York: Guilford Press.

Ellis, A. 1998. *How to Control Your Anxiety before It Controls You.* Secaucus, NJ: Carol Publishing.

Ellis, R. 1999. *Practical Reiki: Focusing Your Body's Energy for Deep Relaxation and Inner Peace.* New York: Sterling Publishing Company.

Enright, R. D. 2001. *Forgiveness Is a Choice: A Step-by-Step Process for Resolving Anger and Restoring Hope.* Washington, D.C.: American Psychological Association.

Epstein, G. 1989. *Healing Visualizations: Creating Health through Imagery.* NY: Bantam Books.

Fanning, P. 1994. *Visualization for Change*, 2nd ed. Oakland, CA: New Harbinger Publications.

Fishman, S. 2000. *The War on Pain.* New York: HarperCollins.

Friedberg, F. 1995. *Coping with Chronic Fatigue Syndrome: Nine Things You Can Do.* Oakland, CA: New Harbinger Publications.

Harp, D., and N. Feldman. 1996. *The Three-Minute Meditator: 30 Simple Ways to Unwind Your Mind and Enhance Your Emotional Intelligence,* 3rd ed. Oakland, CA: New Harbinger Publications.

Hay, L. L. 1999. *You Can Heal Your Life.* Santa Monica, CA: Hay House.

*The Holy Bible: King James Version.* 1982. Nashville, TN: Thomas Nelson, Inc.

*So That's Why! Bible: Making Sense of All the People, Places, and Events of the Bible.* 1997. Nashville, TN: Thomas Nelson, Inc.

Hunter, M. E. 1996. *Making Peace with Chronic Pain: A Whole Life Strategy.* New York: Brunner/Mazel.

Inlander, C. B., and P. Shimer. 1995. *Headaches: 47 Ways to Stop the Pain.* New York: Walker and Company.

Kelly, S. F., and R. J. Kelly. 1985. *Hypnosis: Understanding How It Can Work for You.* Reading, MA: Addison-Wesley.

Lehndorff, P. G. 1997. *60 Second Chronic Pain Relief.* Far Hills, NJ: New Horizon Press.

Matheny, K. B., and C. J. McCarthy. 2000. *Write Your Own Prescription for Stress.* Oakland, CA: New Harbinger Publications.

McKay, M., and P. Fanning. 2000. *Self-Esteem: A Proven Program of Cognitive Techniques for Assessing, Improving, and Maintaining Your Self-Esteem.* Oakland, CA: New Harbinger Publications.

McKay, M., and P. Rogers. 2000. *The Anger Control Workbook: Simple Innovative Techniques for Managing Anger and Developing Healthier Ways of Relating.* Oakland, CA: New Harbinger Publications.

McKay, M., P. Rogers, and J. McKay. 1989. *When Anger Hurts: Quieting the Storm Within.* Oakland, CA: New Harbinger Publications.

Olshan, N. H. 1987. *The Scottsdale Pain Relief Program: The Revolutionary Seven Day Drug-free Program to Reduce Pain.* New York: Beaufort Books Publishers.

Potter-Efron, R. 2001. *Stop the Anger Now: A Workbook for Prevention, Containment, and Resolution of Your Anger.* Oakland, CA: New Harbinger Publications.

Roche, L. 1998. *Meditation Made Easy.* San Francisco, CA: HarperCollins.

Roger, J., and P. McWilliams. 1989. *You Can't Afford the Luxury of a Negative Thought.* Los Angeles, CA: Prelude Press.

Rutledge, T. 1997. *The Self-Forgiveness Handbook.* Oakland, CA: New Harbinger Publications.

Sinel, M. S., and W. W. Deardorff. 1999. *Back Pain Remedies for Dummies.* Foster City, CA: IDG Books

Sobel, D., and A. Klein. 1994. *Backache: What Exercises Work. Breakthrough Relief for the Rest of Your Life—Even after Everything Else Has Failed.* New York: St. Martin's Press.

Starlanyl, D. J. 1999. *The Fibromyalgia Advocate: Getting the Support You Need to Cope with Fibromyalgia and Myofascial Pain Syndrome.* Oakland, CA: New Harbinger Publications.

Starlanyl, D. J., and M. E. Copeland. 2001. *Fibromyalgia and Chronic Myofascial Pain: A Survival Manual,* 2nd ed. Oakland, CA: New Harbinger Publications.

Sternbach, R. A. 1987. *Mastering Pain: A Twelve-step Program for Coping with Chronic Pain.* New York: G. P. Putnam.

Taylor, R. R., F. Friedberg, and L. A. Jason. 2001. *Chronic Fatigue Syndrome, Fibromyalgia, Multiple Chemical Sensitivities: A Clinician's Guide to Controversial Illnesses.* Sarasota, FL: Professional Resource Exchange

Taylor, S., and R. Epstein. 1999. *Living Well with Hidden Disability: Transcending Doubt and Shame and Reclaiming Your Life.* Oakland, CA: New Harbinger Publications.

Temes, R. 2000. *The Complete Idiot's Guide to Hypnosis.* Indianapolis, IN: Alpha Books/MacMillan.

Wall, P. D. 2000. Pain: *The Science of Suffering.* New York: Columbia University Press.

Weiss, L. 1999. *Practical Dreaming: Awakening the Power of Dreams.* Oakland, CA: New Harbinger Publications.

Wells, C., and G. Nown. 1998. *The Pain Relief Handbook: Self-help Methods for Managing Pain.* Buffalo, New York: Firefly Books.

Yapko, M. D. 1992. *Free Yourself from Depression: A Self-help System.* Emmaus, PA: Rodale Press.

# References

Bassman, S. W., and W. C. Wester. 1997. *Hypnosis, Headache and Pain Control: An Integrative Approach.* Roselle, IL: American Society of Clinical Hypnosis (ASCH) Press.

Beecher, H. K. 1946. *Pain in men wounded in battle.* Annals of Surgery 123:96–105.

Benson, H. 1997. *Timeless Healing: The Power and Biology of Belief.* New York: Fireside Books.

Brown, D. P., and E. Fromm. 1986. *Hypnotherapy and Hypnoanalysis.* Hillsdale, NJ: Lawrence Erlbaum.

———. 1987. *Hypnosis and Behavioral Medicine.* Hillsdale, NJ: Lawrence Erlbaum.

Carpenter, S. 2001. *A new reason for keeping a diary.* Monitor on Psychology 32(8):68–70.

Cheek, D. B. 1965. Emotional factors in persistent pain states. American Journal of Clinical Hypnosis. VIII(2):100–110.

Cheek, D. B. 1994. *Hypnosis: The Application of Ideomotor Procedures.* Boston: Allyn and Bacon.

Cheek, D. B., and L. M. LeCron. 1968. *Clinical Hypnotherapy.* New York: Grune and Stratton.

Edelstien, M. G. 1981. *Trauma, Trance, and Transformation: A Clinical Guide to Hypnotherapy.* New York: Brunner/Mazel.

Edmonston, W. E. 1986. *The Induction of Hypnosis.* New York: John Wiley & Sons.

Eimer, B. N., 2000a. *Clinical applications of hypnosis for brief and efficient pain management psychotherapy.* American Journal of Clinical Hypnosis 43(1):17-40.

———. 2000b. *Hypnosis for the relief of pain: What's possible and what's not.* Psychological Hypnosis, 9(2).

Eimer, B. N., and A. Freeman. 1998. *Pain Management Psychotherapy: A Practical Guide*. NY: John Wiley.

Elman, D. 1964. *Hypnotherapy*. Glendale, CA: Westwood Publishing Co.

Erickson, Milton H. 1985. *The Wisdom of Milton H. Erickson*. New York: Irvington.

Evans, F. J. 2001. *Hypnosis in chronic pain management*. In *International Handbook of Clinical Hypnosis,* edited by G. D. Burrows, R. O. Stanley, and P. B. Bloom. London: John Wiley.

Ewin, D. M. 1986. *Hypnosis and pain management*. In *Hypnosis: Questions and Answers,* edited by B. Zilbergeld, M. G. Edelstien, and D. L. Araoz. New York: Norton.

———. 1992. *Constant pain syndrome: Its psychological meaning and cure using hypnoanalysis*. Hypnos XIX(1):57–62.

———. 1998. *Rapid eye roll induction*. In *Hypnotic Induction & Suggestion,* edited by D. C. Hammond. Roselle, IL: American Society of Clinical Hypnosis Press.

Ewin, D. M. and B. N. Eimer. 2006. *Ideomotor Signals for Rapid Hypnoanalysis: A How-To Manual*. Springfield, Illinois: Charles C. Thomas Publisher.

Gravitz, M. A. 1988. *Early uses of hypnosis as surgical anesthesia*. American Journal of Clinical Hypnosis, 30(3):201–208.

Havens, R.A. ed. 1985. *The Wisdom of Milton H. Erickson: Hypnosis & Psychotherapy* Vol. I. New York: Irvington Publishers.

Hilgard, E. R., and J. R. Hilgard. 1994. *Hypnosis in the Relief of Pain*. New York: Brunner/Mazel.

Jampolsky, G. G. 1979. *Love Is Letting Go of Fear*. Millbrae, CA: Celestial Arts.

Kabat-Zinn, J. 1995. *Wherever You Go, There You Are: Mindfulness Meditation in Everyday Life*. New York: Hyperion Books.

LeCron, L. M. 1964. *Self-Hypnotism: The Technique and Its Use in Daily Living*. NY: New American Library.

Linehan, M. M. 1993. *Cognitive-Behavioral Treatment of Borderline Personality Disorder.* NY: Guilford.

McCaffrey, M., and C. Pasero. 1999. *Pain Clinical Manual* (2nd Edition). St. Louis, MO: Mosby.

Melzack, R. 1975. *The McGill Pain Questionnaire: Major properties and scoring methods.* Pain 1:277–299.

———. 1996. *Gate control theory: On the evolution of pain concepts.* Pain Forum 5(2):128–138.

Melzack, R., and P. Wall. 1965. *Pain mechanisms: A new theory.* Science 50:971–979.

———. 1982. *The Challenge of Pain.* New York: Basic Books.

Merskey, H., and N. Bogduk, eds. 1994. *Classification of Chronic Pain: Descriptions of Chronic Pain Syndromes and Definitions of Pain Terms,* 2nd ed. Seattle, WA: IASP Press. 210.

Mutter, C. B. 1987. *Hypnosis in psychiatry. In Clinical Hypnosis: A Case Management Approach,* edited by W. C. Wester. Cincinnati, OH: Behavioral Science Center, Inc. Publications.

Price, D. D. 1999. *Psychological Mechanisms of Pain and Analgesia.* Seattle, WA: IASP Press.

Rossi, E. L., and D. B. Cheek. 1988. *Mind-Body Therapy: Methods of Ideodynamic Healing in Hypnosis.* New York: W. W. Norton and Company.

Rosenstiel, A. K., and F. J. Keefe. 1983. *The use of coping strategies in low-back patients: Relationship to patient characteristics and current adjustment.* Pain 17:33–40.

Schafer, D. W. 1996. *Relieving Pain: A Basic Hypnotherapeutic Approach.* Northvale, NJ: Jason Aronson, Inc.

Seligman, M. E. P. 1975. *Helplessness: On Depression, Development, and Death.* San Francisco: Freeman.

Spiegel, H., and D. Spiegel. 1978. *Trance and Treatment: Clinical Uses of Hypnosis.* New York: Harper Collins/Basic Books.

Stern, C. 1996. *Gates of Repentance: The New Union Prayerbook for the Days of Awe.* New York: Liturgy Committee of the Central Conference of American Rabbis.

Sullivan, M. J., and J. L. D'Eon. 1990. *Relation between catastrophizing and depression in chronic pain patients.* Journal of Abnormal Psychology 99:260–263.

Turk, D. C., and T. E. Rudy. 1992. *Classification logic and strategies in chronic pain.* In *Handbook of Pain,* edited by D. K. Turk, and R. Melzack. New York: Guilford Press. 409-428.

Wall, P. D. 2000. *Pain in context: The intellectual roots of pain research and therapy.* In *Proceedings of the 9th World Congress on Pain,* edited by M. Devor, M. C. Rowbotham, and Z. Wiesenfeld-Hallin. Seattle, WA: IASP Press.

Watkins, J. G., and H. H. Watkins. 1997. *Ego States: Theory and Therapy.* New York: W. W. Norton.

Zarren, J. I. 1996. *Ethical issues in how we identify ourselves as therapists who use hypnosis.* New York Society for Ericksonian Psychotherapy and Hypnosis Newsletter 10(1):6–7.

Zarren, J. I., and B. N. Eimer. 2002. *Brief Cognitive Hypnosis: Facilitating the Change of Dysfunctional Behavior.* New York: Springer Publishing Company.

While this CD is an accompaniment to this second edition of this self-help book, it stands on its own and can be used without the book. This CD uses Hypnosis to gently guide you into a state of relaxed concentration, awareness and inward focus. It teaches you the listener how to use Self Hypnosis as a coping skill for controlling chronic pain. The informative and pleasant suggestions on the CD are easy to follow, and the soothing and relaxing background music helps to further your experience of relaxation and comfort.

This Hypnosis CD is meant to be listened as often as you like in a safe environment when attention to external tasks is not required. It is designed to expand and improve your ability to control and cope with pain and diminish suffering with repeated listenings to the CD over a period of days. Each time you listen you reinforce your developing pain coping skills. Remember the old adage—practice makes perfect. Well, in this instance, practice makes better.

The CD specifically covers:

- What Hypnosis is

- Pain perception and Hypnosis

- Entering a relaxing state of Self Hypnosis

- Rating and lowering discomfort

- Pain relief and comfort imagery exercises

- Healing imagery

- Therapeutic touch and energy healing

- Comfort transfer techniques

- Instant stress control